16
CD TO CD INTERV.
Tel. requested

Healing
Celebrations

Leonard G. Horowitz, D.M.D., M.A., M.P.H.

Tetrahedron Publishing Group
Sandpoint, Idaho

BY LEONARD G. HOROWITZ

Deadly Innocence

Taking Care of Yourself

Dentistry in the Age of AIDS

AIDS, Fear and Infection Control

Healing Codes for the Biological Apocalypse

Emerging Viruses: AIDS & Ebola—Nature, Accident or Intentional?

History of Medicine

2000 B.C. – Here, eat this root.

1000 A.D. – That root is heathen. Here, say this prayer.

1850 A.D. – That prayer is superstition. Here, drink this potion.

1940 A.D. – That potion is snake oil. Here, swallow this pill.

1985 A.D. – That pill is ineffective. Here, take this antibiotic.

2000 A.D. – That antibiotic doesn't work anymore. Here, eat this root.

2010 A.D. – That root is contaminated. Here, practice energy medicine.

2030 A.D. – Energy medicine is passé. Here, connect directly to God.

—Adapted from *Qigong Newsletter*

DEDICATED TO GOD
AND HIS HOLY SPIRIT OF HEALING POWER;
and to those who give trust, praise, and love to Him,
while forgiving, as He does, our sins.
May this work support the mass awakening of humanity
to the ease with which God delivers
miraculous healings and blessings
to those faithful enough to receive them.

Tetrahedron, LLC

Health Science Communications for People Around the World

Copyright © Leonard G. Horowitz, 2000, 2002

Cover designed by Brian Torvik Design
Manufactured in the United States of America

10 9 8 7 6 5 4 3 2

Library of Congress Cataloging Preassigned
Horowitz, Leonard G.
    Healing Celebrations
    p.   cm.
    Includes bibliographical references and index.
    1. Popular Works;   2. Religion
    —Christianity—Bible;
    3. Health Education   4. Spiritual Healing

Card Number: 00 090697
Additional cataloging data pending.

ISBN: 0-923550-08-9

Additional copies of this book are available for bulk purchases.
For more information, please contact:
Tetrahedron • Suite 147, 206 North 4th Avenue • Sandpoint, Idaho 83864,
1-800-336-9266, Fax: 208-265-2775, E-mail: tetra@tetrahedron.org,
URL web site: http://www.healingcelebrations.com

Second printing

IMPORTANT NOTICE:

The information contained in this book is intended for educational purposes only. It is not provided in order to diagnose or treat any disease, illness, or injury of the body, mind, or spirit.

The author, publisher, and distributors of this work accept no responsibility for people using or misusing the potentially empowering information and revelations in this book.

Individuals suffering from any disease, illness, or injury should, as Hippocrates prescribed, "learn to derive benefit from the illness," contact appropriate health care professionals, and seek God's miraculous healing power through faith, prayer, forgiveness of sin and love as soon as possible.

Contents

Foreword

A great evangelist once said, "There is no limit to what God can do through a man totally given over to Him."

The past year, knowing and working with Dr. Len Horowitz has been an honor. I have seen a man in the refiner's fire, being molded and made into the image of God. Yet, at the same time, he has maintained such childlike faith, that if God said it, he believes it.

Being Jewish, he is very aware of his heritage, heir to the great King Solomon. But I see a young David, a man willing to take on Goliath, yet a tender boy after God's own heart. A man willing to change, willing to press towards the high calling that God has on his life. Not the road most traveled, or the road most profitable, but the way that pleases God. He seeks to be a God pleaser, not a man pleaser. How many of us can say that in honesty.

A year ago, if pressed in the wrong direction, some might say Dr. Horowitz had quite a temper. Six months ago he was somewhat able to control himself as the airline representative told him all of his luggage was lost. He was due to speak in two hours and to be the speaker for a four-hour video shoot. There he stood, with no suit, no shoes, no presentation slides, just a t-shirt, jeans, and the sneakers he was wearing. He had every reason to be upset, and was initially, but was able to calm himself after awhile.

Today I spoke with a man that explained to me that love, God's love, is the only way to go! No anger, just love, even when anger seems justified. . . . The man I spoke with today was not the same Dr. Horowitz I met a year ago.

What started the transformation of a high tempered, radical, antigovernment activist? It started on the inside, he had heart surgery by the chief surgeon who is not a practicing physician. He is the great physician—God almighty! The outward manifestation of the inward change is occurring *daily*.

He became a new man (2 Corinthians 5:17). Follow closely, and you shall see a man like the evangelist spoke of a hundred years ago. For a man given over to God can speak the oracles of God in confidence and assurance because his heart is fixed on Him.

Dr. Horowitz is a prophet in the making. The word says, (2 Chronicles 20:20) "Believe the prophet and you shall prosper." I know I have through his teaching, by his example, and from reading this book. You will also!

Dr. Horowitz, we love and appreciate you.

Valerie Saxion*

* Valerie Saxion, N.D., is one of America's most articulate champions of nutrition and spiritual healing. A twenty year veteran of health science in the natural foods arena, she is the co-founder of CSI Inc., a highly successful manufacturer and distributor of nutritional products with a focus on oxygenation. Dr. Saxion co-developed with Dr. Horowitz "Healing Celebrations Unlimited," an international healing ministry, and largely inspired this book. The mother of seven healthy children, Valerie contributes greatly to Christian charities and to feeding the hungry.

Introduction

"No eye has seen, no ear has heard
and no one's heart has imaged
all the things that God has prepared
for those who love Him."

1 Corinthians 2:9,
The Complete Jewish Bible

One half of the world's population should soon be dead according to government officials, authoritative projections, and religious scholars alike. Will you, your family, and friends be among the survivors or the deceased?

Today, people all around the world, including your family and friends, are sick and ailing. A variety of new plagues have struck planet earth, that, according to leading experts, have no known origin or cure. The new plagues include myriad autoimmune system disorders and bizarre cancers that have occurred among people with no family history of such illnesses. Virtually nonexistent before the 1950s, cancers which include lymphomas, leukemias, sarcomas, melanomas, and others are suddenly in epidemic proportions. According to public health authorities, one out of every two Americans are projected to get cancer sometime during their lives. Besides these, contaminated blood and vaccine related disorders are plaguing every nation. The short list of these illnesses includes: chronic fatigue immune dysfunction, or CFIDS, fibromyalgia, lupus, multiple sclerosis, or MS, Guillain Barré, amyotropic lateral sclerosis, that is, ALS or Lou Gehrig's Disease, chronic crippling rheumatoid arthritis, adult and juvenile type I diabetes, and more. Asthma, hay fever, and allergies, that we had to some extent years ago, are rapidly increasing epidemics. They have also been linked to the violation of God's law to keep human blood clean. The relationship between contaminated blood supplies, vaccines, and the current and coming plagues was adequately revealed in my bestselling book, *Emerging Viruses: AIDS & Ebola—Nature, Accident or Intentional?* and my audiotape, *Horowitz "On Vaccines,"* published in 1997 by Tetrahedron Publishing Group (1-888-508-4787). Moreover, the horrific effects childhood vaccinations have had on delivering epidemics of ear infections, attention deficit disorders (ADD), autism, hyperactivity, and sudden infant death (SIDS), to hundreds of thousands of youth is unGodly.

Moreover, people are being intoxicated in ways very few can even fathom. Contaminated air, water, foods, and soils, added to toxic environmental chemical exposures, is taking a dramatic toll on public health. Most diseases today originate from multiple sources, also known as "multifactorial."

In recent years, for example, bizarre upper respiratory infections have became pandemic. During summer, not flu season, hospital emergency rooms were filled to capacity with people experiencing flu-like symptoms. In the Winter of 1998, an unprecedented percentage of the entire North American population developed a chronic upper respiratory infection that would not respond to traditional medical care. The plague increased by January 2000 so that even mainstream newspapers reported it. People were coughing, sneezing, had sinus headaches and congestion. It became chronic, lasted weeks, and was entirely unlike typical viral flus. People were generally not bed ridden, but the disease gnawed at most victims for six, eight, ten weeks or more. Chronic fatigue was a common symptom of this illness. People felt run down. Repeated trips to family physicians for antibiotics often failed to produce long-term benefits. Some felt a little better for a few days as antibiotics killed off secondary bacterial infections, but the primary infection(s) came back.

Most suspiciously, mainstream purveyors of medical propaganda remained silent in the face of the early epidemic. Public health authorities at the Centers for Disease Control and Prevention (CDC), and others elsewhere, who take advantage of virtually every opportunity to dramatize their work and worth, remained silent.

Meanwhile, naturopathic physicians and herbalists, who applied common sense, rational judgement, and God's natural healing modalities, were successfully curing these patients. In natural healing centers it was determined that this chronic upper respiratory infection was most likely related to fungal infections. The simple fact was that when most patients took their body temperatures, they had no fevers. Unlike a viral flu, or bacterial infections, body temperatures remained LOW!

Typically, bacterial or viral infections induce a fever—a body temperature higher than 98.6 degrees. This chronic respiratory disease was associated with lowered body temperature—below 98.6. Thus, naturopaths concluded they were likely dealing with a respiratory fungal infection, and that was why, they reckoned, their patients would not respond effectively to traditional antibiotics. In fact, it was noted that drug therapies, of every kind, actually made many people worse. Antibiotics, besides killing off essential resident microbes that help maintain health through the assimilation of essential nutrients from foods, acidified people's bodies turning their "terrains" acidic. This prompted further fungal growth and recurring illnesses.

Fulfilling Bible Prophecy

Spiritually, according to the scriptures, we shouldn't be surprised by any of this. All the above is actually Bible prophecy being fulfilled. From the "end times" prophecies in Daniel to the pestilence and plagues discussed in Revelation, all of these epidemics are related to contemporary Babylon violating the word of God. The current and coming plagues were heralded by virtually every prophet who blessed the face of this planet. Revelation implicates those who "fornicated with the Devil" and "stole the blood" of God's people. In deceiving world leaders and the "wealthiest merchants," a select few are making vast fortunes from humanity's suffering. Oddly, these people also fund world "depopulation activities."

In fact, the same pharmaceutical industrialists, and international blood "banksters" that I exposed in *Emerging Viruses: AIDS & Ebola*, are implicated here as well. The Rockefeller family, after all, takes center stage in American medicine, world pharmaceutics, and world blood trading.

In the Bible, those who prompted God's wrath, and the great plagues, practiced "sorcery." In *Strong's Concordance*, this word stems from "pharmacopoeia" or pharmaceutics. How fitting for the Rockefeller family, who along with a handful of other political notables, created a monopoly over American medicine and the cancer industry early in the twentieth century. Together with the Royal Family who owned the lion's share of General Motors, or GM, and Alfred P. Sloan, the president of GM, the Rockefellers funded cancer virus research and development long before people ever heard the words "cancer virus." It is no wonder the word "beasts" found in Revelation, associated with the plagues that would destroy half the earth's population, derives from the Greek term that includes "little beasts"—such as those associated with global pandemics such as AIDS and mad cow disease.

This book, thus, heralds the fulfillment of Bible prophecy, not only in the frightening sense, but also in the celebratory sense. *Healing Celebrations* reflects on contemporary health care and contrasts medicine with natural health maintenance and spiritual healing practices. It leaves you with a choice to make—"which will you choose?"

"Come out of her, my people, . . . that ye receive not of her plagues." (Revelation 18:4)

In this book, God's *words* and *laws* are advanced and discussed in testimony to the natural healing spiritual renaissance that is increasingly obvious and uplifting people around the world. Miraculous healings for those who have eyes to see the truth, and ears to receive His good news, are readily available.

Given all of this, I believe it is now critical that you consider what to do to prepare your "temple of God" for the current and coming plagues. I believe you need to take personal responsibility for your health care now more than ever, keeping in mind a spiritual perspective during this extraordinary time in human history. In the coming chapters, I will address the most important things that you can do to boost natural immunity against infectious agents, and get rid of these relatively easily to recover or remain healthy.

The solutions I will present include a five-step process for bringing yourself back to optimal health and then maintaining it. Regardless of whether or not you've ever been intoxicated, vaccinated, exposed to infectious agents, sick, or even "dying," at the present time, you want to do at least the first three of these five steps. If you are sick and ailing with any of the immune system related disorders or cancers mentioned above, or other chronic diseases, you will want to perform steps four and five as well. To repeat, the first three of these five steps should be done by everyone. After completing the first three, if you are still sick, you should go on and do steps four and five under the care of a professional that embraces a wholistic approach and natural healing methods.

These five steps for achieving, maintaining, or regaining optimal health include:

1) detoxification,

2) deacidification,

3) boosting your immune system every way possible—
   physically, mentally, emotionally, socially,
   environmentally, and above all, *spiritually*,

4) oxygenation therapies, and

5) bioelectric therapies.

All of these steps are intimately related to spiritual healing as you will shortly learn. Especially the last two steps.

In the final chapters of this book the "Scriptural Correlates and Antecedents for Health" are presented. These chapters, I feel, include the most vital knowledge of our time. It is written here to empower you with God's love for your healing and protection. Especially the protection of your children who are also His.

For me, this research and development has been an unimaginable gift that I am blessed here to share with you. I pray that you will be likewise blessed by the nature and Spirit of this contribution.

Forever in the Spirit of health,

Leonard G. Horowitz, D.M.D., M.A., M.P.H.

Chapter 1.
Sacred Wisdom for Healing

"May God grant to me to speak properly,
And to have thoughts worthy of what He has given;
For it is He that guides wisdom and directs the wise.
For in His hand are we and our words,
All understanding and knowledge of trades.
For it is He that has given me unerring knowledge of what is,
To know the constitution of the world
and the working of the elements. . . .
The powers of spirits and the designs of men,
The varieties of plants and the virtues of roots;
All that was secret or manifest I learned,
For wisdom, the fashioner of all things, taught me."

The Wisdom of Solomon 7:16-20,
The Apocrypha

This book is a glorious celebration of the beneficence of God being poured out on humanity at this unique and challenging time in history. This glory becomes obvious in the revelations that people have been receiving, not only from the Bible, but also from the Holy Spirit. More and more people throughout the world have, in recent months, perceived extraordinary increases in their spiritual sensitivities. Synchronous experiences have occurred far more regularly than ever before. For example, you think about something special, you begin working on a project, and all at once, miraculously, these thoughts manifest in your life. Positive results seem to flow out of you, and into you, like never before. Work goes smoothly. The next contacts you need to make in your life suddenly become apparent and present. You just happen to turn the radio on, and there is a message you need to hear! You turn the corner and there in the store widow is the book you need to read! You synchronously open the book to the exact page and sentence containing the message you longed to receive. You open your Bible in the morning and, *ditto*, God gives you the perfect lesson for your day. Little miracles, and big miracles alike, are happening for you routinely. And when they do, you simply "thank God."

It is wonderful to be living in God's realm—the Holy Kingdom. And if you're not there yet, just wait. Extraordinary blessings are in store for you should you choose to get on track.

That's what this book is about—"Healing Celebrations." There is God's way of healing and there is the "sorcerer's" way of healing. The later, the pharmaceutical industrialist's way of healing, is infinitely inferior to God's Divine Way. God's way of healing doesn't include popping a pill to cure every ill. God's way of healing is so totally miraculous, and so simple, that it has been overlooked and suppressed by the purveyors of drugs and pharmaceutical propaganda.

The Wisdom of Solomon

God's way of healing and maintaining health, which is all Biblically prescribed, begins with developing the "Wisdom of Solomon"—a virtual manual on the dynamics of human development and Godly spiritual functioning:

> For [wisdom] teaches self-control and understanding,
> Righteousness and courage;
> Nothing in life is more useful to men than these. . . .
> Because of her, I will have immortality.
> She penetrates and permeates everything, because she is so pure;
>
> For she is the breath of the power of God . . .

passing into holy souls, generation after generation.
For the Lord of all loves her. . . .
She is initiated into the knowledge of God.
(Solomon 7:24-27; 8:3-4; 8:7-8)

Wisdom dictates that health must be addressed wholistically—physically, mentally, emotionally, socially, environmentally, and above all *spiritually*. That's God's way of caring for the blessed being you are. You are, after all, a Holy child of God, created in the image of your Father. You have been endowed with the elements and skills to make you a masterful co-creator of health and positive physical realities, including love in your family and peace on earth. Of course, all this begins with you.

The blessed "Prince of Peace," better known as Jesus of Nazareth, more correctly called Rabbi Yeshua—the Son of God, actualized an everlasting healing ministry called Christianity.

The name "Yeshua" is best used because it was the Messiah's Hebrew name. Literally translated it means "God saves." You will learn later why the *sound* of the *word*, Yeshua, is powerful.

Contained in God's two covenants is a contract to protect, prosper, and co-create enduring health for His faithful followers. That is, people with eyes to see and ears to hear His truth are to be blessed. Yeshua, better than any, exemplified the healing power and creative practice of applied faith in the Holy Spirit. "Seek first the Kingdom of God," Yeshua advised, and then "all else will be added unto you." (Matthew 6:33; Luke 12:31) This also included physical health and everlasting spiritual life. Thus, the context of healing includes physical as well as spiritual dynamics. The entire field of electromedicine, as will be discussed later, best exemplifies this union of healing elements. How Yeshua, for instance, was able to touch people, and miraculously bring about healing, even as they touched his clothing, is an important question. The answer lies in the Divine vibe—the Holy Spirit—which comes through an electromagnetic matrix or grid. The

3

science and documentation supporting this thesis is advanced in my previous book, *Healing Codes for the Biological Apocalypse* (Tetrahedron Publishing Group, 1999).

The knowledge drawn from the new Bible code revelations discussed in *Healing Codes for the Biological Apocalypse* includes the essence and importance of the Holy Spirit for healing, which like Solomon's wisdom, "penetrates and permeates everything."

As Apostle Paul prescribes in 1 Corinthians 14:12, it is most important to seek understanding of these spiritual matters, and "especially what will help" to uplift the knowledge and wisdom of God's children. In this regard, he instructed, " I couldn't talk to you as spiritual people but as worldly people, as babies, so far as spiritual matters are concerned. . . . Now the natural man does not receive the things from the Spirit of God—to him they are nonsense! . . . But the person who has the Spirit can evaluate everything, while no one is in a position to evaluate him." (1 Corinthians 2:14-3:1)

To know God, and your essence, you have to know the Spirit. You need to understand that spirit is an electromagnetic phenomenon. In other words, the Holy Spirit includes electromagnetic frequencies that empower healing. This is what allows God's love to pour out through you, and generate miraculous healings. It is God's electromagnetic technology being transmitted to you, and through you. Though this concept may be foreign to you, science has determined that the entire universe is permeated by electromagnetic fields—energy matrices. The whole universe is a spiritual frequency grid.

Experiencing the Holy Spirit within you, is your God given right and inheritance. You were created in the Father's image with his spiritual constitution and certain creative potentials. Included here is the potential to create health and healing. In essence, you have been blessed with the Holy Spirit. You can

4

think of this as an electromagnetic matrix of creative potential or Divine possibilities. When you have *faith* in the Father and *trust* His laws, words, covenants, and the wisdom behind these, then whatever is in your heart to create that is good will manifest "on earth as it is in heaven." In other words, if your purpose is pure, that is, in service to Him and His children in some loving, meaningful, and/or spiritually uplifting way, then He will cause it to bear fruit.

Having your Holy Spirit pour out to people, by your loving, sharing, and caring for others, is perhaps the greatest purpose in life. It is the fabric that binds humanity together, raises, uplifts, and connects our spirits and brings mankind closer to Godkind. When you have that happening for you, it is because you have placed your will in line with your Father's will to serve others in a meaningful way. Then the potential to produce miracles arises naturally by grace.

By projecting the image of what you desire, with faith and trust in God, it will be miraculously and spontaneously created. This occurs through your words, articulated in prayer. These sounds transmit powerful messages into the electromagnetic matrix of the Holy Spirit, that embodies love and creative potentials. God does the rest.

In essence, you are a miracle co-worker, created by God to serve others.

I give you this knowledge in advance, because when it comes to celebrating your Divine healing power, everything you do short of recognizing your Divine connection, your spiritual gift to produce miracles as a holy empowered child of God, will be inadequate for your higher calling. Conversely, if you really want to bathe in the glory of God, the Divine waters of universal sustenance, you must immerse yourself with faith and trust in your prayer power to manifest the miracles from within you through the Holy Spirit.

In Matthew 18:3-4, Yeshua said, "Yes! I tell you that unless you change and become like little children, you won't even enter the Kingdom of Heaven! So the greatest in the Kingdom is whoever makes himself as humble as [a] child."

Education: The Inner Process

The Greek root word for "education" is "educare," meaning "to draw forth from within." The process begins before we were born and largely impacts the destinies of children.

Before a presentation I recently gave in Denver, Colorado, a boy, eight years old or so, walked up to me and said, "Dr. Horowitz, I was vaccinated when I was an infant, and I almost died. My parents were afraid I would die, but I pulled through. I know there are many others who aren't so fortunate. Thanks for your vaccine work, and not being afraid to tell the truth."

My response was, "Guess what? You were saved because God has a great purpose for you, just like every single one of us. We're all on track for fulfilling humanity's destiny. Each of us has a unique role to play in the great healing; a piece to place into the great puzzle of the Messianic Age. I'm glad to see He spared you so you can contribute your wholeness and wellness to the world."

Years ago, as a Harvard graduate student, when I first began to research healthy human development, and educational applications for children, I developed and published in the scientific literature the "Self-Care Motivation Model." I wanted to determine what it would take for a child, like this young boy, to become a self motivated and self reinforcing agent for his own healthier and happier human development. I set out to find the key requirements—the vital lessons that would get children excited and committed to evolve into more successful human beings. Ultimately, God blessed me with the plan which came from a third grade class, "right out of the mouths of babes."

The "Self-Care Motivation Model" diagram is provided in figure 1.1, and associated with this is a "Wholistic Model" diagram seen in figure 1.2. These diagrams provide an overview of what comprises a human being, and how our individual parts function to actualize a greater whole. Figure 1.1 diagrams the dynamics of intelligent behavior in relationship to God's values. Figure 1.2 provides a view of our human composition, and how these various parts connect you to God's Divine Spirit. These diagrams, and the knowledge and wisdom reflected in them, provide a virtual owners manual for managing our Godly temples. They provide a guide to healthy human development and spiritual evolution.

As it was in the days of Solomon, so it is today. The Holy Spirit is being poured into your "temple of God," and God wants you to build your temple as beautiful, pure, and wholesome as possible. God wants you to fully understand your composition, and your Divine essence, and care for these majestic gifts, as much as possible, to pay Him tribute. Then, by grace, you will receive His greater blessings including His miracles.

This lesson appears critical to your survival in the twenty-first century. That is, to defend yourself against the current and coming plagues, you need to make sure your temple remains pure and Divinely empowered.

Counsel of "No Fear"

Before examining the different parts of these diagrams, I want to return to the boy in my audience again. His double reference to fear, once again, brings King Solomon's great wisdom to mind. You see, Solomon's wisdom was largely gained from his father's counsel. When, for example, it came time to build God's great temple, King David counseled Solomon (1 Chronicles 22:11-14) saying, "My son, . . . may God be with you and give you common sense and understanding, . . . so that you will observe the laws of God. Then you will succeed, if you take care to

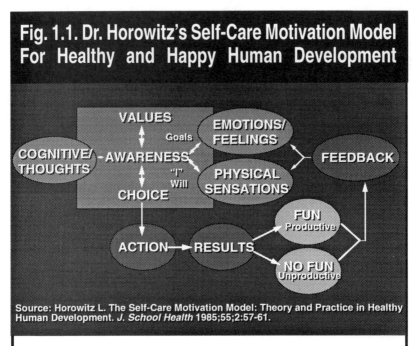

Fig. 1.1. Dr. Horowitz's Self-Care Motivation Model For Healthy and Happy Human Development

Source: Horowitz L. The Self-Care Motivation Model: Theory and Practice in Healthy Human Development. *J. School Health* 1985;55;2:57-61.

Figures 1.1 and 1.2 provide the key elements of "self knowledge" to understand human behavior and spiritual "cybernetics"—feedback systems related to healthy and happy human development. Source: Horowitz, LG. The Self-Care Motivation Model: Theory and practice in healthy human development. *J School Health* 1985;55;2:57-61.

Fig. 1.2. A Wholistic Model of Human Beings

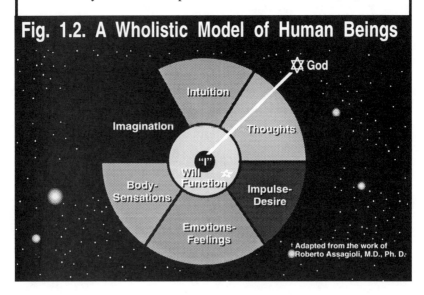

† Adapted from the work of Roberto Assagioli, M.D., Ph. D.

obey the[se] laws and rulings . . . Be strong, be bold; don't be afraid or become discouraged! "

So Solomon was warned not to be afraid of the darkness surrounding his calling to obey God's laws and build the Lord's temple. David's counsel was based on the realization that as soon as you enter into fear, you lose your connection to the matrices of the Holy Spirit, and the electromagnetic magnificence of God's peaceful and loving universe. Peace and love is God's domain. As soon as you allow yourself to entertain fear, whether it's fear of an illness, such as cancer, or fear of a person, group, or nation, you lose your connection!

Wise counsel includes turning your fears over to God, blessing them, and blessing as well the object(s) of your fear(s). Finally, you need to forgive the people whom you fear, because, as you will learn later when I share the spiritual significance of forgiveness, this returns you to the Holy Spiritual domain of God. Then you recover your Divine power to co-create health and healing, not only for yourself and your family, but for this entire planet.

Thus, King David's counsel to Solomon in preparing him to build God's temple included the wisdom of "no fear," and to follow God's laws.

Taking Your First Steps

Believe it or not, you already have everything you need for optimal health, happiness, success, prosperity, career enrichment, and life fulfillment. As figure 1.2 diagrams, you have an incredible mind, body, emotions, imagination, intuition, and powerful "will" to make positive choices for better health and living. You maintain a spiritual nature, a Holy Spirit, which automatically empowers your state of well-being. It's up to you to use your innate endowment for the benefit of all. You have the ability to constantly experience love, create happiness, be productive, and fulfill your greatest goals. It's all a matter of choice, and the choice is yours right NOW! It's actually easy once you learn the basics beginning with understanding God's values and how they relate to your own values.

Values, very simply, are close cousins to emotions and feelings. Unless you are mentally ill, your values reflect your desire to avoid pain and gain pleasure. Likewise, God's laws, His "Ten Commandments," are predicated on the wisdom that pleasure, associated with values like health, happiness, prosperity, and love, is preferable to pain, fear, and loss. God's covenants rely on this wisdom in that God places faith and trust in His children to abide by His commandments. These relay His values. Therefore, by avoiding the "sin" of violating His laws, you will naturally avoid the harsh judgements—the pain, fear, and loss that sin generates.

If you simply begin by clarifying values you will develop a firm foundation for general lifelong learning, health, and success. If you have children, start by teaching them to appreciate the value of health, love, joy, and prosperity. Everything that God wishes to give every one of His faithful children are His *values.*

Hippocrates, the great grandfather of modern medicine, once said, "Health is among the greatest of human blessings." This is apparently why Yeshua spent so much of his time producing miraculous healings. He knew that people would be highly impressed after witnessing extraordinary recoveries. Divine faith, he reckoned, might be best inspired in people witnessing Divine healings. He rightly, of course, gave all the credit to God. His principle instruction was clear and powerful: "[S]eek first His Kingdom and his Righteousness, and all these things [health and all other blessings] will be given to you as well." It was not by accident the very next words he spoke focused on the demon of fear. "Don't worry about tomorrow, tomorrow will worry about itself." (Matthew 6:33)

Recognizing that health is among the greatest of human blessings and Divine values, if you simply align your values to God's values, you'll start *Healing Celebrations* on the right foot. If you are uncertain as to how important health is to you and your family, just ask yourself, "What would happen, or what would it cost me, if I lost my health. How much pain versus pleasure might I endure?" Moreover, if you want to know God's values, simply read the Bible. Throughout the old and new testaments, health is cited numerous times as a value God commits to protect for you, and instill in you, so long as you obey *His* laws. Otherwise, as in the Book of Job, He pulls His protective hand away to authoritatively demonstrate His power, and lovingly prove His covenant.

Goal Setting

After establishing the value of health, as seen in figure 1.1, you should set your health and healing goals.

It has been said that a principle reason why people fail to set or achieve their health goals is because subconsciously they are self-defeating. Decades of psychological research suggests that previous traumas affecting self-esteem, and self-image, underlie such self-destructive conditioning and patterning.

However, here I am relaying the wherewithal to produce miracles. Rather than strenuous psychoanalysis and/or arduous behavioral therapies, *Healing Celebrations* directs your attention, acknowledgment, and *faith* to the Heavenly Kingdom wherein instantaneous recovery is available. In fact, as prophetic minister Kenneth Copeland announced during his nationally televised program recently, faith in Yeshua, and his blood sacrifice, effectively washes away ancient memories upon which self-destructive behaviors rest. So instead of seeking expensive psychotherapy first, he and I recommend faithful prayer first and always.

After examining your health values, and setting your healing goals, list your first, second, and third most valued desires and why you feel so strongly about acquiring them. Meditate and pray on these as your most precious goals to be achieved. In God's Holy Kingdom, wherein time and space is relative, *they are already achieved*! Therefore, to see them manifest, visualize them daily while focused in the Holy Spirit, and call them into current certainty through sincere greatful prayer.

While you're at it, endeavor to determine your unique purpose in life. What heartfelt yearnings inspire you? Everyone longs to be helpful and productive in some meaningful way. Actualizing your purpose, your unique contribution to others, builds self-esteem and the love of God. Both of these factors certainly promote health.

Are there any social service crusades to which you long to subscribe? The Bible says an investment seeded into the Gospel returns a hundred fold. Clarify and set personal goals for life-long fulfillment based on this knowledge, inspiration, and motivation. With a little self-discipline you'll achieve more than you ever dreamed possible.

Taking Action

Once your health and healing goals have been set, prayerfully articulated, and documented in your *Healing Celebrations* diary (following the index), develop an action plan based on priorities. In other words, develop a step by step action plan to achieve your goals. Record in your diary what you will need to have, do, or be, to manifest your dreams. For every difficult step or requirement, seek mentors or experts in the field to emulate or consult. There's no need to reinvent any wheels. Do what successful people are doing and you will succeed. Your individuality will automatically be expressed along the way.

For example, let's say you suffer from chronic fatigue, poor circulation, lowered body oxygen levels, and respiratory distress. Your highest priority might be to stop smoking. It would make sense to quit as soon as possible. You would need to establish an action plan to quit. Pray for your next step. From God's Holy Kingdom you will receive guidance. The right instructor, or perhaps the perfect smoking cessation program, will synchronously manifest in your life to help you achieve your goal.

Personal Awareness Training

Figure 1.2 also shows that as a human being, your components include physical, mental, emotional, imaginative, and intuitive parts, as well as a "will" center of self-awareness and choice-making that, ideally, is in tune with your spiritual nature. In Hosea 4:6, God said that His people are destroyed for lack of applied knowledge. Your self knowledge, and how you relate to God, and His Holy Spirit within you, is key to your health and everlasting life.

Therefore, I encourage you to develop your personal awareness and self-observation skills through your "will" center. This will permit you to take stock of your physical, mental, emotional, imaginative, and intuitive behaviors. God always speaks to you through one or more of these channels if you "have the ears to hear." Translation of His language comes through these components, if your listening skills are enhanced and you attune yourself to be sensitive.

To begin your personal awareness training for healing, assess your intra-personal assets and liabilities. Which of these parts of you are optimally healthy? Which are imbalanced; over or under-utilized? Analyze and upgrade your inventory to support your health, happiness, and greater stress-free productivity in keeping with God's highest callings for you.

Mental Health Challenge

You may have mental blocks which routinely keep you from achieving a state of productive bliss. Your mind has thoughts, and distractions, including unproductive fears and concerns. The voice in the back of your head—what some people call your "internal dialogue"—can drive you crazy with anxiety, which for God is a "sin."

The root word for "sin" stems from the Greek archery term meaning "off the mark." Your arrows, or actions, miss their target, and veer away from God's grace when you sin. That is, you've made choices inconsistent with God's laws and productive plans for you. Allowing your internal dialogue—your undisciplined mind—to drive you to drink is such a "sin."

In this regard, I am reminded of the story relayed in *The Complete Jewish Bible* in Matthew 14:26-33, wherein Yeshua instructs regarding the need for peace of mind and trust in God:

> When the apostles saw him [Yeshua] walking on the lake, they were terrified. "It's a ghost!" they said and screamed for fear. But at once Yeshua spoke to them. "Courage," he said, "it is I. Stop being afraid. Then Kefa called to him, "Lord, if it is really you, tell me to come to you on the water." "Come!" he said. So Kefa got out of the boat and walked on the water toward Yeshua. But when he saw the wind, he became afraid; and as he began to sink, he yelled, "Lord! Save me!" Yeshua immediately stretched out his hand, took hold of him, and said to him. "Such little trust! Why did you doubt?" As they went up into the boat, the wind ceased. The men in the boat fell down before him and exclaimed, "You really are God's son!

Later in Matthew 17:17 and 17:20, Yeshua cautioned his students again regarding the incapacitating affect of fear and distrust on healing and other miracles. "Perverted people, without any trust!" he scolded, "Because you have such little trust! Yes! I tell you that if you have trust as tiny as a mustard seed, you will be able to" move mountains.

It is that little jabbering ego voice that strains to comprehend the miraculous reality available to you. It's this same voice that trusts little, worries much, and asks survival-linked questions, such as "How will I pay these huge bills?" It distrusts the supernatural means of manifesting prosperity to miraculously pay and/or cancel your debts. In other words, it rarely considers, or *trusts*, your Divine nature and capacity to manifest miracles at every moment. It lacks faith in God and in your Holy Spirit. That's precisely why you need to become aware of this self-defeating part of you. Learn to observe this immature voice, override it when it issues self-destructive, fear-based, sinful messages, and give it over to God for disciplining if you're having trouble directing it yourself.

Most people have, in fact, caught themselves thinking negative thoughts, and substituted positive ones for better outcomes. This is one small, but vital, example of the powerful need to master your mind, body, emotions, imagination, and intuition—the subordinate parts of yourself—by asserting your "will" to consistently choose for your, and God's, highest good. Otherwise, it will be as though you're left adrift in the wind blown turbulence of Satan's sinful sea.

Body and Emotions

Body sensations, emotions, and feelings should also be understood for their primary spiritual function. God created you, like every other natural creation, according to a *cybernetic system* in keeping with His natural laws of balance and judgement. Cybernetics is defined in *Webster's* as "a system of feedback and communication in all living and nonliving systems."

What an incredible concept! "Feedback and communication" is present in every living and nonliving God creation. God created this entire universe to operate within a system of feedback and communication so that everything would maintain homeostatic balance, that is, peaceful existence and/or coexistence.

As a Holy child of God, you were also designed with cybernetic feedback and communication systems. That's the principle function of emotions, feelings, and body sensations. God gave you these so that when you make choices, and take actions, your body sensations, emotions, and feelings give you (often immediate) internal feedback as to whether or not you are acting in keeping with His laws, values, and goals for you. These feedback circuits inform you whether or not you are on the right track to achieve, or maintain, your positive health values, goals, and blessings.

As seen in figure 1.1, based on your highest values and goals, you choose to take action(s). Actions produce results. Results provide feedback. In keeping with natural cybernetic laws, this feedback comes to you in two forms: positive or negative body sensations, and emotions and feelings, that is, pains or pleasures. This, again, relates to values, especially God's values, whereby God always wants you to feel good, manifest health, and produce miracles. That's His covenant with His people who follow His directions. Sin produces the opposite—you ultimately feel bad, lose, manifest disease, become dysfunctional, and produce little of value.

An example of this is overeating. If you stuff your face, even when you know you shouldn't, how do you end up feeling? Pretty lousy. As seen in figure 1.1, life turns painful or nonproductive when you make poor choices. In other words, "no fun." This feedback comes in the form of body sensations, like the pain and stuffiness in the pit of your stomach, and negative feelings and emotions as you beat yourself up for your masochistic actions. Relatedly, your mind condemns you by saying, "What's the matter with me? I knew I shouldn't have done that!" Naturally, the cybernetic results taste rotten as it comes back up, feels rotten if it stays in, and smells even worse if it isn't eliminated fast! The ultimate irony is that God created you as a potentially magnificent human being capable of creating miracles, and you're doing yourself in, then feeling lousy about yourself because of it.

This rips at the heart of your self-esteem and "self-love"—not "self-love" in the narcissistic sense, but in the heartfelt appreciation for the miraculous being that God created you to be. You need to forgive yourself and ask Him to forgive you for your transgressions against yourself and Him. As Exodus 32:6 and 1 Corinthians 10:7 proclaims, people who over-indulge in food and drink, as idolaters, are sinning before God.

Let it go, forgive yourself, but repent. Stop doing yourself in. This is the purpose and function of personal awareness training. To get back on track, tune into, with heightened awareness, your emotions and feelings, your mental thoughts, your body sensations, and God's Holy Spirit. These will give you feedback to motivate your turn from self-destructive ways—the essence of repentance—to become healthier, happier, and more successful in life as a self-motivated and self-reinforcing agent for your own personal development in service to God and His people.

Your "Will" to Produce God's Wonders

Once again, at the center of this dynamic cybernetic feedback process is your "will." It is capable of observing your body sensations, thoughts, feelings, imaginative visions, and intuitive insights. It is your center of self awareness and choice making. Obviously, if you can observe, evaluate, and even regulate the subordinate parts of yourself, you are greater than the limitations posed by any of them. It is your "will" center of self awareness and choice making that enables you to master yourself, transcend liabilities, and further develop your positive attributes.

Moreover, if you align your personal will with your spiritual will, then miracles are facilitated. It is likely that your unique spirit, or soul, has a special destiny to fulfill. So that if you align your personal will, and the choices you make, with your spiritual will that's aligned to God, then guess what? Miracles naturally result along with an ongoing series of synchronicities that guide you to fulfill your unique destiny. That's when you experience yourself as "in the flow." This is what the Bible refers to in Psalms 37:23 where you are told, "If the Lord delights in a man's way, he makes his steps firm." Also, Psalms 85:12 reports, the steps of men in right standing with God are blessed with prosperity and guidance. Here the Bible says, "The Lord will indeed give what is good, and our land will yield its harvest. Righteousness goes before him and prepares the way for his steps. Proverbs 16:8 also says, "In his heart, a man plans his course, but the Lord determines his steps." And finally, Proverbs 20:24 asserts that, "A man's steps are directed by the Lord."

So if you align your personal "will" center of self awareness and choice making, with your higher spiritual will, and that is likewise aligned to God's will for you, then your steps will be ordered by God to consistently move in the direction of health and prosperity. That's God's covenant with His children, as you will later learn in more detail. Then miracles occur routinely in your life, because there is nothing stopping their flow. These are readily available in God's magnificent Kingdom which is fully miraculous. That is, His Holy Kingdom thrives on miracles. So that's what the potential is for you to enjoy.

In summary, you should endeavor to develop optimal self-awareness, self-regulation skills, and a spiritual dependence on God. Develop your strength of will and power of choice so that you can co-create your fate. Your steps will be ordered by God. By affirming your power to control your sinful urges, and the intra-personal dynamics that keep you stuck—especially negative thoughts—you will help God guide you to the "promised land." Shape your social outcomes by asserting your "will" with the intent to serve Him, heal yourself, and be helpful to others.

Use your personal power to master the challenges you face each day.

Progress is made one day and one step at a time. Progress may appear slow but is forthcoming. Nurture the virtue and value of patience. Always take action based on your highest good and greatest goals. Act consistently in support of these, in your best interest, and for the purpose of nurturing your own, or other people's personal development and spiritual growth.

Turn conflicts into opportunities by realizing the perfection in every situation, and in all of life. When problems arise, ask yourself, "What's good about this problem?. . . What's not ideal yet? . . . How can I make it more ideal, and how can I have fun doing it?" Always seek to determine your role in co-creating and resolving conflicts.

Each "crisis" is an undeniable "opportunity." Remember, you can choose to see every glass as half empty or half full. Above all, always pay special attention to the feedback you receive following your choices and actions. These are like God's voice, given to you, to redirect your steps toward success. Negative social experiences, likewise, are co-created for a purpose, and always by choice. To remain healthy, happy, and productive, your personal choices must comply with a higher purpose, spiritual order, and/or God's will, in order to maintain and uplift your personal power to love and serve. Painful experiences are, therefore, opportunities for better health, living, and decision making. Take responsibility then for every negative you experience. Learn to resolve each problem by assessing your role in co-creating it, then take affirmative action for correcting it.

Always be grateful, thankful, and forgiving. God's universe is forever giving. All living and nonliving systems are constantly empowered, revitalized, and rebalanced just for the sake of being. Unconditional love reflects this same power in each of us. You are capable of giving, and worthy of receiving, unconditional love. With this, the entire force of the universe supports you and your cause. Thus, be eternally grateful for everything you have, for all your gifts, abilities, and possessions. Start each day by giving thanks, and praising God, for all of life's (big and little) blessings.

Finally, when in doubt, if you stumble or fall, offer your difficulties to God for resolution and clarity. He will forgive you for wrongdoing if you simply ask for forgiveness. Likewise, forgive yourself and others for any past wrongs and/or harm you may have suffered at the hands of the ignorant or unGodly. You lose yourself in the present by being angry and/or resentful about the past. That's not God's way, that's the way of the bruised ego. Every moment is an opportunity to experience life anew, and create it to be the way your heart desires. As Winston Churchill said, "Free will and predestination are identical." With God's help, you have extraordinary power to let go of your traumatic past and choose a brighter future. Give thanks for this awesome power and all your possessions. God gave you everything you have. You may have worked hard for it all, but without God's hand in it, you'd never have been so blessed.

Chapter 2.
Preparing Your "Temple of God"

"Go to the ant, you sluggard;
consider its ways and be wise!
It has no commander, no overseer or ruler,
yet it stores its provisions in summer
and gathers its food at harvest.
How long will you lie there, you sluggard?
When will you get up from your sleep?
A little sleep, a little slumber,
a little folding of the hands to rest—
and poverty will come on you like a bandit
and scarcity like an armed man."

Proverbs 6:9-11,
The Holy Bible

Preparing your "temple of God," wholistically, to combat the current and coming plagues, as well as celebrate miraculous healings, is what you will entertain next. This process depends on five important steps. These include: 1) detoxification—a step that includes fasting, 2) deacidification—changing your body chemistry to make it more alkaline and less acidic, 3) boosting immunity every way possible. This includes the wholistic approach to total well being that I already mentioned including physical, mental, emotional, social, environmental, and above all spiritual correlates and antecedents for health and healing, 4) oxygenation and related therapies, and 5) bioelectric therapies including spiritual healing practices. This chapter details the first of these vital steps—detoxification and fasting.

Step 1: Detoxification

If you're like most people, eating foods loaded with white flour, refined sugar, man-made oils, genetically engineered proteins, chemical preservatives, and various food colorings, your body is like a waste disposal ripe for the growth of bacteria, viruses, funguses, and cancer cells. This risk poses a major threat to the onset of most modern diseases. You need to open up your eliminative channels to get rid of the garbage—this toxic waste—you have been storing mostly in your liver and fat cells.

Fasting

"Here is the sort of fast I want," said the Lord in Isaiah 58:6-11. His counsel advised fasting so that every area of your life will be free. Your spirit, mind, and body are included so that no disease will come upon you! Fasting, God said, facilitates your Divine freedom. "Your light will break forth like morning . . ." and your "healing shall spring forth speedily." Your fast, God declared, will even right your relationship with Him! So that He can go before you, and the glory, His goodness, will be your guardian.

My earlier audiotape programs, *Horowitz "On Healing,"* and *Taking Care of Yourself*, explain how fasting can detoxify your body, give your organs a rest, and bring natural healing by cleansing your body of toxins. Fasting can even help reverse aging processes. By fasting only three days a month, you can help rebuild your immune system to help fight off infectious illnesses and degenerative diseases. Sickness may simply reflect an overloaded immune system—one burdened by exposures to toxins of various kinds.

Length of Fasts

In general, three to nine day fasts are recommended for health and longevity. It is a scientific fact that by fasting three days a month, you will heal faster, and may extend your life several years. A three day fast helps rid your body of toxins, a five day fast starts the healing process, and a ten day fast should take care of most problems before they begin.

Fasting Caveats

- Don't fast on water alone!
- Don't chew gum or mints. This starts the digestive juices flowing and is harmful to your system.
- Don't eat junk, especially during a fast. The last thing you eat will be the next thing you crave! If you eat junk, you'll want more junk. If you eat veggies, you'll want something healthy. Your body is designed by God to want healthy food, but when you eat the wrong things, you deaden your senses to what is right. Then your body no longer knows what to crave.
- Don't drink orange or tomato juice on a fast.

Preparing For and Beginning Your Fast

To prepare for your fast, eat only raw, preferably organic, foods for two days.

On the third morning, on an empty stomach, drink one 8 oz. glass of *Clustered Water*.* Studies show that *Clustered Water* dramatically increases the absorption of anything you take orally around the time you drink it. Thus, absorption of nutrients is aided, along with the cleansing and replication of cellular structures. 20-30 minutes later, drink 1 oz. of *OxyAdvantage*™* to further aid in the detoxifying process.

Before eating lunch, on an empty stomach, take a second 8 oz. glass of *Clustered Water*, then wait a half-hour before having a second 1 oz. serving of *OxyAdvantage*™.

*All products mentioned in this section will be discussed in detail later.

G.I. Flora Pro

I also highly recommend a product called *G.I. Flora Pro*™. Without friendly bacteria populating your digestive tract you could not survive. In fact, a balance of at least 85% helpful bacteria to 15% potentially harmful germs is required to optimally assimilate the nutrients from your diet. Your health and energy is dependent upon this assimilation and symbiotic relationship with gut natural soil-based microbes. Unfortunately today, particularly due to antibiotic overuse, few people maintain this healthy gut flora balance.

G.I. Flora Pro™ contains psyllium husks and soil-based micro-organisms (SBOs) that were originally in food. SBOs are highly resistant to stomach acids, and they are capable of implanting, surviving, and metabolizing throughout your intestinal tract. These bacteria colonize your gut to help reduce pathogens. Active ingredients include microbes from the families: Bacillus, Arthrobacter, Azotobacter, Pseudomonas, Aspergillus, Chaetomium, Streptomyces, Trichoderma and Verticillium that all work to assist your body in establishing an optimal intestinal flora. These extra strength microbes make *Lactobacillus acidophilus* and *Streptococcus* organisms, that people commonly consume as supplements, seem weak by comparison.

G.I. Flora Pro™ organisms also work by releasing enzymes that help neutralize toxic chemicals in your system. They help assimilate food from macronutrients to micronutrients. Combined with *OxyAdvantage*™ this often reduces or eliminates constipation, diarrhea, and other digestive disorders. Periodic enemas, as I will mention shortly, are also recommended for optimal intestinal and digestive function.

Beginning on day three of your fast, you should take two 600 mg. capsules of *G.I. Flora Pro*™, with 8 ounces of water, mid-morning; another two at night before retiring. Half this dose is recommended for maintaining colon health after you're through fasting.

Taken as directed, *G.I. Flora Pro*^{TM} microbes are extremely aggressive against pathological molds, yeast, fungi, and viruses. More powerful than other gut treatment products, this patented proprietary blend is developed using organic growth factors that enhance the SBOs ability to perform under stress and varied toxic conditions. Highly resistant against thermal, chemical, and other digestive stressors, *G.I. Flora Pro*^{TM} provides the right microbial mix for disease prevention, immune support, and health enhancement.

Water and Juice Recommendations for Fasting

Every day drink about half your body weight in ounces of water. For example, if you weigh 150 pounds, drink 75 ounces of water a day. Health science consensus currently believes that steam distilled water is best for fasting, while alkalinized water is the best for maintenance hydration. (More on this later.) Steam distilled water actually goes in and pulls out toxins from your organs. It literally pulls out the mire that gets caught in the follicles of your colon that breeds disease.

You will also find that drinking steam distilled water helps curb your appetite, unlike a sweet drink or juice that causes your body to want more.

When on your fast, dilute your pure juices with steam distilled water. Again, do not drink orange or tomato juice on a fast. The best juices are fresh lemon, cabbage, beet, carrot, celery, grape, apple, and green drinks made from leafy green vegetables. These are excellent detoxifiers.

Raw cabbage juice is known to help heal ulcers, cancer, and all colon problems. However, it must be fresh, not stored. It loses its vitamin U content if stored for too long.

Another excellent blend is the juice from three carrots, two stalks of celery, one turnip, two beets, a half head of cabbage, a quarter bunch of parsley, and a clove of garlic. This could be one of the best juices on our planet for healing many illnesses.

The "Master Cleanser" Juice Fast

Another favorite juice preparation is Stanley Borroughs's "master cleanser." This is especially good for alkalinizing the body and raising body temperature to help resolve infections and flu-type illnesses.

Here's how you make and use it:

Take a gallon jug and fill it 3/4 full with steam distilled or other pure water. Next, squeeze the juice of 4-6 fresh lemons and add it to your gallon jug. Third, add grade B or C maple syrup (available from your health food store). The lower the grade, the less refined and more packed with trace minerals and other nutrients. At this point, you should have a delicious 100% natural lemonade. Finally, add cayenne pepper—the hottest cayenne pepper you can get. Most cayenne is around 30,000 to 40,000 heat units (H.U.) Try to get at least 90,000 H.U. If you can find it, get African Bird cayenne pepper which is as high as 180,000 H.U.! Add as much cayenne as tastes good to you, and then add a pinch more. In other words, add as much cayenne as you can comfortably tolerate. I typicaly use about 2-3 teaspoons full of the 90,000 H.U. cayenne per gallon, or a bit more as my stomach and taste dictates.

Make a gallon of this every day and drink it for 9 days. This "master cleanser" should be used for no more than 10 days.

On day one of the "master cleanser" fast, here's what happens: You begin to get hunger pangs. Your stomach is used to being filled with food. You've become habituated to eating, so you get hunger pangs. Every time you get a hunger pang, drink some more "master cleanser." This, I guarantee, will take away your hunger pangs. By the end of the day, you should have finished the entire gallon of "cayenne-spiked" lemonade.

By day two, you will notice that you aren't that hungry anymore. Don't forget that you are drinking as much of this stuff as you can comfortably tolerate. You begin detoxing, cleansing your system, and by the second day most people don't feel too hungry.

By day three, you may be shocked because you are now, not only, *not* hungry, but you are beginning to feel better and more energized. I've had Olympic class athletes tell me that after three or four days on the "master cleanser," they were so energized, they were able to run marathons. It's totally surprising how well your body can do without food. You'll notice that you will start feeling a lot cleaner and lighter by day three.

Detoxification headaches may come. Drink additional water to remove toxins from your bloodstream. It may help to add a little *OxyAdvantage™* for this as well.

By day three, you'll look in the mirror and notice that your skin is starting to get clearer, brighter, and younger looking. You're getting rid of some of those wrinkles; and you're seeing magic happen before your eyes. These miracles are coming about from simple detoxification. So you basically want to do this fast for at least 3 days.

Other Juice Fasting Tips

Pure vegetable broths, with no seasonings added, are also good for fasting. To prepare these, gently boil veggies, including onions and garlic, for 30 minutes. Two to three times a day drink the juice from these blended or strained broths.

Watermelon fasts in season, or fresh carrot or grape juice, also make fine fasting juices.

If you must eat something, have a slice of watermelon (in season). Always eat watermelon alone. Alternatively, organic grapes, or fresh apple sauce made with the skins on and processed in a blender or food processor is satisfying and won't significantly disrupt your fast.

Use oat bran on your fast. It helps cleanse the colon by adding fiber. It is best to take this at night before going to sleep.

Spirulina can also be used during a fast. It is loaded with protein and all the vitamins and minerals your body needs.

Enemas

Enemas during a fast are an absolute must. Enemas during fasting will assist your body in its cleansing and detoxifying effort by washing out all the toxic wastes from your alimentary canal. Enemas should be taken at least once, preferably twice a day. (Upon rising and before going to bed.) One pint to one quart of lukewarm distilled water is sufficient. Enema bags, including instructions, are available in any drug store.

Fasting Results

Fasting brings the body back to doing what it was designed to do, accomplish the will of God without the hindrances of fatigue, obesity, and illness. Most people, following initial withdrawal from chemical dependencies (including caffeine and sugar) see and feel a dramatic difference in their health status by day three of a good fast. People commonly feel lighter and more energized and notice improvements in complexion and eye color. These changes indicate you are on track for *Healing Celebrations.*

Maintenance After a Fast

Always break fasts gently with high quality, fresh, and organic foods that are minimally processed. This is essential to maximize the benefits of your fast. After fasting, your body is like a sponge and you need high quality materials to build high quality cell structures.

In the realm of whole raw organic foods, and related products, is the pleasant tasting and smooth green drink I developed for my family. It's called *Green Harvest*™. This whole raw organic food supplement will help in both continued detoxification as well as immune system boosting. Directions on the container advise how you can make a delicious fruit smoothie and a meal replacement with *Green Harvest™*. I recently fasted for forty days on primarily *Green Harvest™* fruit smoothies, vegetable broths, and occasionally water melon.

Likewise, I continued to use *Clustered Water* and *OxyAdvantage™* daily, and occasionally took *G.I.Flora Pro™*, to maintain my gut flora.

Another powerful aid in rebuilding your immune system is Pau d'arco and Echinacea tea mixed with one-third unsweetened cranberry juice four times a day.

Lightly steamed veggies in their broth with whole grain brown rice can be added slowly to end your fast, and used as part of your maintenance diet.

Colon Cleansing

If your waist line is expanding or you are carrying a tire around your waist that hangs over your belt, it's probably not your stomach that has expanded, but your colon that is ballooning, packed with old fecal matter. If your bowel movements come out like a tube of toothpaste, you may have as much as thirty feet of your large and small intestines literally packed with old fecal matter. If you eat three times a day and have bowel movements less than once a day, you need to start cleaning out your colon. You can start by incorporating a psyllium based product into your diet. You can find psyllium husks at your health food store.

Stir a teaspoon of psyllium into good water or juice, and then drink the mixture. The psyllium turns into a Brillo-pad-type of substance—a fiber that moves through your gut and cleans out your intestines. Along with enemas, it pulls out waste stuck to your colon wall. This will help you become more regular.

Liver Cleansing

An excellent way to stimulate the liver to detoxify is with coffee enemas. These are most often recommended for metabolic cancer therapy, and are extremely helpful in many detoxification programs. These enemas are given for stimulation and detoxification of the liver, not for cleaning your intestines. The coffee is absorbed directly through your colon wall. It travels via the portal vein directly to your liver which, in turn, produces bile.

This detox method could initially cause nausea, which in small amounts is desirable, but if too great, reduce the amount of coffee used, or use the enema on a full stomach. The coffee should be stronger than for drinking, and not diluted.

Coffee enemas are believed to alkalinize the first part of the intestines, enhance enzyme function, and stimulate the production and release of bile. They do tend to deplete potassium levels, however, and therefore must be used with proper diet or supplementation.

The coffee enema procedure is as follows: Mix 2 tablespoons of ground (drip) coffee, neither instant or decaffeinated, with 1 quart of steam distilled water heated to body temperature. Fill your enema bag with two cups. Do this twice daily. Take this enema preferably on your knees, or lie down on your back, legs drawn close to your abdomen. Breathe deeply while the enema is going in. Retain the fluid for 10 to 15 minutes.

To detoxify in serious conditions, take two coffee enemas per day for two weeks. Then reduce these to only one per week for one month.

Your body may have a buildup of toxins from time to time. Common symptoms indicating toxicity include decreased appetite, headaches, fatigue, and general malaise. If these occur, increase coffee enemas once again to one per day for a maximum of three to four days wherein symptoms should improve or disappear. Then return to a healthier routine.

Liver Dysfunction Diet

This diet must contain high-quality protein, such as white turkey meat, leg of lamb, game, white low-fat cheese, yogurt, cottage cheese, goat's milk, sprouted seeds and grains, raw nuts (especially almonds), and sesame butter or ground sesame seeds sprinkled over food, raw and steamed vegetables of all kinds.

Small frequent meals are preferred rather than two or three large ones. Raw fresh vegetables and fruits, free of artificial colors, preservatives, and chemicals of any kind, are a must.

Avoid all animal fats, canned and refined foods, synthetic vitamins, drugs, strong spices, sugar, coffee, black tea, and alcohol.

The best juices at this time are carrot/celery/parsley with one teaspoon of cream for every eight ounces of juice. Red beets are excellent. Cucumber, papaya, blue grapes, lemon, and green juices are also good.

The best herbs for liver dysfunction include St. John's wort, lobelia, parsley, horsetail, birch leaves and sarsaparilla. Rosemary can help stimulate the liver to produce more bile. Marigold supports the liver in purifying blood. Lilac has been used to decongest livers. Olive tree leaves facilitate the discharge of gallstones. Dandelion is recommended to help reduce liver inflammation.

The best teas for liver health include peppermint, spearmint, chamomile, and thyme.

Additional Ways to Detox

You can eliminate toxins through your secondary detox organ, your skin. So sweating is an important aspect of the detoxification process. Exercise, sweat lodges, and saunas—particularly steam saunas—are great. There's even a portable steam sauna available that administers essential oils to stimulate detoxification.

When you exercise, you are moving your extremities, and pumping your lymphatic fluids. The lymph is required to get rid of toxins in your body. Lymph massage techniques also help promote proper lymphatic drainage as you are detoxifying.

Another way to cleanse your lymph system is to incorporate dry skin brushing. Get a body brush that you never intend to use in the shower, and put it aside for brushing your entire body upon waking up in the morning. This will help your body shed layers of built up dead skin. This dry skin brushing, and avoiding synthetic materials that keep your skin from breathing, will also aid in the oxygenation process which is essential in attaining and maintaining optimal health.

Herbs and *Rose Tea*

One of the most important aspects of the detoxification process is to cleanse your liver and bloodstream. The liver, besides your skin, is your primary detoxification organ. It is like the oil filter of your car. It helps clean the blood of chemicals and other toxins encountered in the modern world. So, it makes sense to pamper it a bit. A multitude of detoxifying herbs and their formulas can help with this cleansing process.

One great product, for example, is called *Rose Tea*. It assists both the kidneys and the liver in purging toxins. It's a special formula of 10 herbs which specifically cleanse your body of much of this accumulated debris. In fact, detoxifying with *Rose Tea* is such an important first step that I recommend you detox with this tea for at least a week, drinking 2-3 cups a day, *before* you take any *Green Harvest*™—the food supplement I mentioned earlier and will discuss in greater detail ahead.

The following herbal ingredients found in *Rose Tea*, and description of their effects, can give you a pretty good idea about the power of herbs to detoxify your body:

Dandelion Leaves (*Taraxacum officinale*)—Contains glycosides, triterpenoids, potassium, beta-carotene, and silica. These provide powerful blood cleansing and strong diuretic effects. Dandelion leaves help the function of the liver and aids the flow of bile. Due to its diuretic action it is very helpful to use to overcome water retention and toxin elimination.

Violet Leaves (*Viola odorata*)—Contains alkaloids, saponins, flavonoids, and salicylate. This herb is used to aid the respiratory system. It effectively removes toxins from your chest area. It also helps remove inflammatory toxins from your kidney and bladder.

Honey Suckle (*Loniceraw flos*)—An astringent that helps remove toxins from the digestive tract.

Rose Hips (*Rosa canina*)—Contains vitamin C, pectin, and carotene. Rosehips provide a good natural source of vitamin C, which in megadoses, can help the immune system fight off viral infections, colds, and the flu.

Marigold (*Calendula*)—Contains carotenoids, saponins, flavonoids, and phosphorus. Calendula is a great blood cleanser. It works by removing toxins from your circulatory and digestive systems. It also has powerful healing properties.

Sage Rubbed (*Salvia officinalis*)—Contains flavonoids, salvene, and pinene. It is also high in calcium, magnesium, manganese, silicon, sulphur, traces of iron and zinc, triterpenoids, and camphor. It also helps remove toxins from the respiratory system.

Panax Ginseng (*Araliaceae*)—Contains glycosides, ginsenosides, antioxidants, selenium, copper, manganese, cobalt, and biotin. Ginseng is beneficial in many aspects of health. It is particularly helpful in treating general weakness, exhaustion, and depression, and is famous for its aphrodisiac affects.

Horsetail Powder (*Equisetum arvense*)—Contains silicon, glycosides, organic acids, and selenium. It is high in calcium, potassium, and magnesium. It helps balance the nutrients in the kidneys.

Nettle Leaf (*Urticae dioica*)—Contains glucoquinine, formic acid, and vitamin C. It has great general cleansing and strengthening properties. It works to remove toxins from the blood.

Cleavers (*Galium aparine*)—Contains glycosides, gallo-tannic acid, and citric acid. It works with the lymphatic system to detoxify the skin and gastrointestinal tract.

Besides *Rose Tea* to help eliminate toxins from your body, the majority of poisons in your diet can be eliminated by incorporating more fresh fruits and vegetables.

Chelation Therapies

Many people are turning to chelation therapies as well as herbs for detoxification. Chelation, like oxygenation and bio-electric therapies that are discussed later, is another largely suppressed, yet proven effective, method for detoxifying your body. You can use chelating agents to get rid of harmful metals, metabolites, and free radicals. Chelation agents can be taken orally or administered intravenously by health professionals.

Chelating agents bind with heavy metals such as lead, mercury, and cadmium—toxins that enter your body through water, food, vaccines, dental amalgam fillings, etc. Chelating agents bind these metals to facilitate their elimination from the body through the urine. Once heavy metal toxins are eliminated from your body, nutrients in your diet are better able to work constructively to promote health and healing.

Chelation therapies are commonly recommended in the treatment of circulatory problems such as atherosclerosis and gangrene. The chelating agents attach themselves to, and help dissolve, the plaque blocking your blood vessels and blood flow.

Other diseases that may be alleviated or cured by chelation therapies include Parkinson's, Alzheimer's, arthritis, and multiple sclerosis.

"Despite reservations voiced by many in the medical establishment," writes medical physician James Balch in his *Prescription for Nutritional Healing* (Avery, 1997), many severely disabled, high-risk individuals have reported dramatic improvement in arterial circulation after chelation treatments.

Fig. 2.1. Chelating Nutrients and Their Uses

Nutrient	Recommended Dosage	Indications
Alfalfa liquid or tablets	Double the amount recommended on the label	Increases oxygen availability to help prevent oxidation of cells and tissues.
Apple pectin and Rutin	As directed on the label.	Liver detoxification and body alkalization. Chelates and removes toxins from the body.
Calcium	1,500 mg daily.	Replaces lost calcium due to chelating agents. Use the calcium citrate form.
plus Magnesium	700 - 1,000 mg daily.	Displaces calcium in cells of artery wall.
Coenzyme Q_{10}	60 - 90 mg daily.	Benefits circulation, reduces blood pressure, and promotes chelation.
Garlic (Kyolic)	2 capsules twice daily with meals.	A good detoxifier and chelating agent.
L-Cysteine and L-methionine	500 mg each twice daily on empty stomach. Take with juice or water. Do not take with milk. Take with 50 mg vitamin B_6 and 100 mg vitamin C for better absorption.	Two of the most helpful natural dietary chelators.
L-Lysine plus Glutathione	500 mg each daily.	Helps to eliminate toxins and heavy metals. Effective free radical scavengers and antioxidants. *Caution*: Do not take lysine longer than 6 months at a time.
Selenium	200 mcg daily.	A strong free radical scavenger.
Vitamin A	25,000 IU daily. If you are pregnant, do not take more than 10,000 IU daily.	Aids in excretion of toxins. Use emulsion forms for easier assimilation.
plus Natural beta-carotene or Carotenoid complex	25,000 IU daily. As directed on the label.	
Vitamin B complex plus Vitamin B_3 (niacin) and Pantothenic acid (vitamin B_5) and Vitamin B_{12}	100 mg 3 times daily. 50 mg 3 times daily. 50 mg 3 times daily. 200 mcg 3 times daily.	Protects the body from toxins and improves cellular functions. *Caution:* Do not take niacin if you have liver problems, gout, or high blood pressure.
Vitamin C complex with Bioflavonoids	5,000 - 15,000 mg daily in divided doses.	Powerful immunostimulants and chelating agents.
Vitamin E (d-alpha only)	Begin with 600 IU daily and increase to 1,000 IU slowly per day.	Eliminates toxins and free radicals. Emulsions are assimilated more easily and safely at higher doses.

Adapted from: Balch JF. and Balch PA. *Prescription for Nutritional Healing, Second Edition.* New York: Avery, 1997, pp. 540-542.

Chelating agents are widely available through health food stores, drug stores, and herb shops. These include: alfalfa, rutin, fiber, and selenium; combinations of calcium and magnesium chelate with potassium; formulas containing chromium, pectin, garlic, and potassium; coenzyme Q_{10}; iron, sea kelp, and zinc chelate.

In addition, figure 2.1 lists various nutrients that are believed to be safe and effective as chelating agents when taken as directed by your health professional.

Homeopathics for Detoxification

Homeopathic remedies are another excellent tool to assist your body in eliminating heavy metals. These have also been shown to reverse some of the symptoms associated with vaccine injury.

As a dentist, people often ask me about mercury toxicity associated with dental amalgam fillings. I learned about this problem in the early 1980s when serious research began to prove that mercury, one of the most toxic substances on earth, was leaking out of dental amalgams. In 1982, I stopped using mercury amalgam fillings in my dental practice, but I still needed to help many of my patients detox. For this I turned to homeopathics and it most often worked well.

Homeopathic nosodes have also been used successfully in reversing the damage caused by vaccines. Frankly, anything you can do to assist your body in the detoxification process is good for vaccine injuries as well.

As this chapter details, there are myriad ways of detoxifying your body ranging from the simple and inexpensive to the more elaborate and costly therapies. My advice, generally speaking, is try the natural, time tested, inexpensive modalities first.

Chapter 3.
Deacidifying Your "Temple"

"Do you not know that your body
is a temple of the Holy Spirit, who is in you,
whom you have received from God?
You are not your own;
you were bought at a price.
Therefore honor God with your body."

1 Corinthians 6:19
The Holy Bible

Deacidification, or simply alkalinizing your body, is the second most important self-care strategy you can employ to guard yourself against the current and coming plagues. Here again, you'll see why I've recommended the tried and true detoxification technique known as the "master cleanser" (see Chapter 2)—the inexpensive mix of fresh natural lemonade and cayenne pepper.

The "master cleanser" has the ability to alkalinize your system to a pH of around 7.5—the pH most people need to feel vibrant and healthy. Both cancers and funguses thrive in people whose body pH is significantly lowered by risky lifestyles. They become intoxicated, acidified, and infected. Most pathogenic forms of bacteria, viruses, funguses, and cancers can't grow in an alkaline environment, so they simply die out.

Today, one main reason so many people are suffering and dying is because of the proliferation of funguses in their bodies. What causes these fungi to grow? *Funguses can only thrive and proliferate in an acidic environment.* When your body is encumbered with excess toxins and acid, they have a perfect breeding ground. As mentioned in my introduction, why my colleagues and I suspect an increase in upper respiratory infections is because of mycotoxicity—fungal infections associated with a drop in body temperature, not a fever which is indicative of bacterial and viral infections. That's why these flu-like illnesses resist antibiotics. Symptoms may improve somewhat after taking antibiotics for a couple days as secondary bacterial infections resolve; but the chief problem—a residual primary fungal infection—persists, and the symptoms often return.

Cayenne pepper, once again, not only helps raise body temperatures, which is helpful against these illnesses, but it deacidifies your body as well. In fact, besides being called the "Roto-rooter of cardiovascular systems," because of cayenne's ability to help dissolve harmful cholesterol plaques, this red hot pepper is one of the most alkalinizing substances you can consume. Bacteria, viruses, funguses, molds, and according to scientific consensus, cancer cells have a very hard time growing in a cayenne alkalinized body.

So if you keep your body slightly more alkaline, generally speaking, opportunistic fungal infections, and the little bacteria and viral "beasts" associated with the prophesied plagues in Revelation, pose little threat.

Body Chemistry, Nutrition, and Optimal Health

Very simply, your body is an electrochemical creation. If "you are what you eat," then the nutrients that you absorb, and how efficiently you absorb them, determines your health through chemical as well as electrical pathways. These dynamic processes all relate to body pH. In other words, acid/alkaline balance in your body affects bioelectrical reactions occurring in every cell, and every tissue, at every moment.

Body pH is the acid/base balance of your body and its tissues. Generally speaking, depending on the organ or body fluid tested, a healthy adult's pH should be between 7.3 and 7.6. In children's tissues, their pH should be between 7.4 and 7.5. When the pH drops from this, disease rapidly ensues. For example, if your pH dropped to 7.0 you'd be in a coma. If it went below 7.0, you'd probably have a heart attack. Locally, cancer cells typically grow in a pH of 4.0-4.5. In fact, pH balance as low as 6.0 to 7.0 in some organs predisposes them, and you, to various chronic illnesses.

Again, "if you are what you eat," then you would expect nutrition to play a vital role in your body chemistry, pH, and general health. Today's typical "Western diet" grossly short-changes people in their nutritional requirements for health. The amount of living foods you would need to consume to maintain the proper pH balance of your body, for example, is about 85% living vegetables. That is, you would need to rearrange your schedule, virtually your entire life, to prepare meals consisting of about 85% fresh organic vegetables. So your best bet is to do the best you can and consume mostly pesticide free vegetables and fruits. Moreover, if you can't get live *organic* vegetables, then make certain that you wash your produce very well in a nontoxic soap (such as Dr. Bronner's) using a thorough rinse. Then, from these vegetables, make your fresh juices. Because in these juices are not only the nutrients, and the special combination of minerals that only nature can provide from good soil, but also electrical components you need to thrive.

Bioelectric Properties of Cells and Foods

Very simply, within the cells of every carrot, piece of lettuce, or apple you consume are electrical charges. These electrical charges are commonly called "electrons." When you eat food, you are actually consuming an electrochemical mixture of nutrients. Just like fruits and vegetables, every cell in your body maintains a negative electrical charge across its outer membrane. Foods are generally positively charged and, because of this, are attracted by, and pulled into, the cells. Most noticeably, the alkaline minerals like sodium, potassium, calcium, and magnesium are all positively charged. These are called "electrolytes," or "electron loving," because of their positive charge and their propensity to be attracted and absorbed by oppositely charged cell membranes. In other words, electrons transfer across cell membranes attached to these minerals, just as they do across gold, silver, copper, and other metals.

Many people don't realize that calcium is a bonafide metal listed in the metals section of the periodic table of elements. It is also the most dominant charged material as it travels across cell walls. The best source of calcium in the food kingdom is your fresh dark green leafy vegetables, and NOT MILK! Calcium citrates and calcium gluconates, NOT CALCIUM CARBONATES, are your best forms for supplementation because their chemical nature simulates having been predigested. They are already bound to amino acids or chelated for increased absorption. Natural chelation commonly occurs when plants produce structures that are readily absorbed into human cells.

You probably don't know that by simply chewing on fresh green grasses, swallowing the juices and spitting out the fibrous pulp, you can survive in the wild without rations. The fresh grass juice supplies the proper pH, alkalinized minerals, and other essential nutrients required for life. The fact is, no one should ever starve when lost in the woods. This simple knowledge can help save lives.

Understanding the bioelectric and biochemical relationships of your body to pH changes, can be additionally life saving. For example, concerning heart attacks, which commonly occur in association with a drastic drop in blood pH, cayenne pepper once again has its miraculous place. If you place a little cayenne pepper under the tongue of someone who is suffering a heart attack, you can literally save their life. That heart attack generally is caused by electrical signals not getting to the proper heart muscles. By adjusting their body's pH quickly using cayenne placed under the tongue, the proper blood chemistry and electronics around the heart may be rapidly restored to stop the attack.

Like cayenne pepper, oxygen also alkalinizes the bloodstream and your body. That is, it increases the pH of your blood and body fluids, and supports healing in many ways. The subject and importance of oxygenation for therapy and spiritual health will be addressed in greater detail in Chapter 5.

Cell wall electrolyte balance is largely affected by body chemistry and blood pH. Proper circulation as well as hydration is also dependent on acid/base balance, that is, pH. Many diseases can be easily reversed by simply rectifying body chemistry.

For instance, many asthmatics have been helped and cured by balancing their pH. Asthma's main cause, according to many researchers and clinicians, is dehydration. Disturbed water regulation in the body can predispose to asthma. Water is released through the lungs. This helps regulate blood oxygen as well as fluid levels.

In high altitude clean mountain streams, the water gives off high levels of negative ions. About 1,000 negative ions per cubic millimeter are thrown off every 1,000 feet of higher altitude. The streams on the mountain tops are filled with the hydroxyl ion (OH⁻). These combine with, and help eliminate, harmful "free radicals" in the body.

Aging also is a result of dehydration and lowered pH. Cultures that live, on average, well into their hundreds, typically consume high pH water containing earth's vital minerals. Thus, aging can be defined as "dehydration and an accumulation of acid waste resulting in disease."

Certain foods, as well as waters, can help raise your body's pH. These include the grain millet, a component of the *Green Harvest™*, as well as vegetable juices that deliver a pH in the range of 8.0.

A few low cost products are also available to help raise blood and body pH. These include a product called *Alkalife*. Two drops in an eight ounce glass of water raises the pH from about 7.0 to 8.0. A three month's supply for one person sells for about $20.00 (U.S).

One word of caution: Some people use baking soda to attempt to raise their body's pH, but this can radically upset their sodium/potassium balance. This balance can also be disturbed by the effects of sodium chloride, table salt, on the sodium and chloride balance in their bodies.

Fluids, Deacidification, and Healing

In earlier days, paramedics attending accident victims would immediately run intravenous solutions containing liquid bicarbonate into their bloodstreams, especially if their hearts had stopped. If they didn't, prior to electrically stimulating the heart, the victim would inadvertently pump acid blood back into the heart which would again prompt heart failure. In other words, they could get their hearts pumping electrically, but if the signals couldn't carry across the heart muscles because of the acid environment, patients would be in trouble. Thus, you can see the crucial nature of blood pH.

Although few hospital workers explain, the nutrient drip bags used for pre-op and postoperative patients, is typically a form of sugar water, and *always* a potassium chloride solution. This is done to supply required salt. Of course a wide spectrum sea salt is the ideal supply since table salt disturbs your natural sodium/potassium balance. If you like using salt in your foods, then use raw Celtic (or French) sea salt. This is thought to be among the best. It maintains the correct electrical components. This will help you lose weight as it reduces fluid retention.

Your body works like your car engine. Without the right fluids, your engine fails. Typically if you lose blood or body fluids, then potassium is the number one thing you likely need. You need a three-to-one ratio of potassium to sodium in your system to maintain health.

That's why among the sports drinks on the market today, the leading brands contain potassium as a chief ingredient. The unfortunate thing about most sports (and soft) drinks is that they also contain chemicals and toxic man-made sugars like aspartame. This causes a number of problems. For example, above 86 degrees, aspartame turns to formaldehyde which greatly impairs liver function and health. The liver becomes intoxicated and hardened by such chemical assaults and becomes dysfunctional. This becomes problematic in that proper liver function is required to make the simple sugars necessary for proper brain function.

Given the nature of pH, the acid increase with lowered pH is exponential. This means with pH—"power of Hydrogen," or "potential of Hydrogen"—if you go down the scale, a 6.0 pH is ten times more acidic than a 7.0 pH substance. A 5.0 pH solution is 100 times more acidic than a pH 7.0. A 4.0 pH is 1000 times more acidic than pH 7.0.

As a result of this dramatic increase in acidity with a small reduction of pH, it can take as much as thirty-two glasses of high pH drinking water to compensate for the damage done by one glass of soda pop containing phosphoric acid!

Soft drinks that contain sugar, as well as phosphoric acid, can knock your system for a double loop. Especially if you have consumed these drinks for years. A person in his early forties who perhaps began drinking colas in his teens, is likely to suffer from severe allergies.

Water for Hydration and Detoxification

Nearly everyone, at one time or another, has cleaned a dirty sink. You know what it took—soap and water. But did you know that to clean the grease off the sink, the soap functioned because it was highly *alkaline*. What alkalinity does is change the surface tension of the water to make it more *hydrating*, and far more capable of cleaning and clearing off the debris.

During detoxification, the hydrating and alkalinizing function played by pure water is critical to the cleansing process. During detox, many toxins come out through your skin, more come out through the urinary tract, and still more through your breath, like the steam you see outdoors on a cold Winter day.

International studies show that populations with little or no history of illness, such as cancer, drank higher pH waters. After all potential risk factors were considered and factored out, it became evident that they had been drinking waters with a pH 9.0 to 10.0.

Today, many scientists believe that this is too alkaline. It may cause laxative effects. Water manufactured with such high pH may produce far too many hydroxyl ions. These can act as free radicals and cause cell injuries, cell death, immune system challenges, and even predispose to cancers.

But nature has been balanced by God to circumvent these risks. High mountain streams, where most water sources originate, contain rocks, organic sediment from decaying trees, and naturally chelated ionic minerals. These waters that have the perfect balance of potassium to sodium, and calcium to magnesium, can be powerful health promoters. These chelated waters can actually help a person detox continuously.

Toxins that come from the petrochemical industry are usually, like grease, acidic. Acid waste deposits—fluorides, chlorides, some compounds containing sulfur, and/or phosphorous—require alkalinizing agents to neutralize, clean-up, or detox. Likewise, humans are acid making machines. Lactic acid builds up from the routine use of your muscles. You build up lactic acid even when you're seated watching television or operating a computer. Muscles get sore because lactic acid deposits seep from the muscles like sweat. If you have nothing to carry this acid away, principally alkalinized water, the acids literally pile up in dehydrated muscles and joints and cause musculoskeletal aches and pains.

Bathing with alkalinized water is also great for detoxification. A cup of Epsom salts, or apple cider vinegar, poured into your bath water can really help relax your muscles. What happens is this: When you're in a warm bath, your pores open, and absorb the magnesium sulfate (Epsom salt). In the process, the salt dissolves the lactic acid stuck within the muscles and joints. That's why you feel like a piece of spaghetti when you exit the bath. You may feel a little dizzy at the same time because you just released a lot of these toxins back into your bloodstream. These go to the brain and often cause light-headedness. A large glass of high pH water, in this case, will relieve the symptoms.

If, on the other hand, you don't consume enough good water along with enough minerals from, let's say, sea salt, then you're in for a host of problems from writhing pains to peptic ulcers.

"What is 'good water?'" you might ask. According to James Karnstedt, among the nation's leading experts in the field, he prefers distilled water. "It's clean, and it's pure, and many professionals recommend distilled water," Jim said in an interview I hosted with him for our audiocassette program called, *Survival Water: pH and Oxygen* (Tetrahedron Publishing Group, 1999).

If one chooses distilled water, "there's two schools of thought about it," Jim explains. "One is, make sure you get enough minerals in your diet along with the distilled water. My particular philosophy is, at that sacred moment when water touches your lips and winds its way down into all of your organs, and surrounds your tissues, it is an electrochemical substance. When it's distilled, or treated with reverse osmosis, most or all of the minerals are taken out, and you no longer have the electrical component. That water is no longer conductive. Distilled water does not conduct. So, if there is any way you can get minerals into your water when they go down your throat, then you're drinking something that has a lot more potential vitality to it. . . . If you drink distilled water, there are little mineral concentrate drops that you can put in your pocket or purse and squeeze those into your water to satisfy your need for the electrical component."

Sadly, people everywhere purchase bottled water in *soft* plastic jugs. These present a problem when the bottles are heated above room temperature. Then they leach some of their chemical compound—organochlorines—into the water. This reduces the pH of the water, sometimes dramatically, and presents health risks. If you buy water in *soft* plastic containers, you should transfer the water to glass storage containers as soon as possible, otherwise these toxins may accumulate in your body and cause harm.

For instance, Dr. William Ray, a world renowned pioneer in women's health, clinical ecology, and environmental medicine, found these organochlorines, only available from soft plastic jugs, in the breast tissues of *all* the women he tested that had breast cancer. He concluded that these compounds can be stored in your body and inhibit the proper lymphatic flow to contaminated organs.

Thus, pure high pH water plays a critical role in maintaining health through detoxification and deacidification processes. I can't stress enough how vitally important it is to increase the amount of water you drink. *You should drink about half of your body's weight converted into ounces of pure, fresh, higher pH water daily.*

Eliminating Acid Lifestyle Risks

What causes your body to become acidic are lifestyle risks that are generally promoted through television, radio, and the print media. We've been brainwashed into believing that the garbage we see advertised is actually healthy. During my Master's in Public Health program at Harvard University in behavioral science, health education, health promotion, and media persuasion technologies research, I learned about every consumer behavior. Advertisers study behavior in depth, in advance, and develop messages according to research standards and proven protocols so that you, the consumer, can be masterfully manipulated. In fact, you don't even know how or when you are being manipulated when it occurs. And when you talk about lifestyle risks, the number one risk to humanity, body acidity, must be seriously considered.

What causes your body's chemistry to become acidic are eight primary lifestyle risks. These include: caffeine, nicotine, white sugar, chocolate, alcohol, virtually every over-the-counter drug as well as illegal pharmaceuticals, meat—especially pork and beef, and last but not least, stress.

Interesting enough, almost every one of the above consumables pose a risk to cardiovascular diseases and heart attacks. Body acidity and dehydration, once again, being the principle culprits.

Body acids and toxic wastes accumulate in fatty tissues, your lymph system, and your arteries, in addition to certain organs. According to experts who conducted published studies, because of dehydration, your arteries may develop little "oxidative pits." Natural cholesterol produced by your body then patches these little holes in artery linings. *Dietary cholesterol is not, therefore, the villain effecting heart disease as was once thought, and still generally believed.* The problem begins with your natural cholesterol produced and deposited on your artery walls in order to plug the holes. These little patches are acidic. As such, they naturally attract calcium and form calcium deposits as well. Thus, dehydration, calcification, and cholesterol build up in your arteries are all associated with acid fluids you may be drinking. This reinforces the need for you to be drinking half of your body weight converted to ounces, in good, clean, bioelectrically alive, alkaline water.

Look around and you'll notice that very few people have weaned themselves away from all eight of the acidifying lifestyle risks. It is well known that stress, or at least chronic negative responses to it, has been linked to various illnesses including cancer. But few people recognize the link that meat consumption can have on cancer as well.

Meat acidifies your blood and body tissues, and increases your risk of cancer. Meat and meat-by-products contain their own cell wastes. They contain uric acid even before they are metabolized as food in your body. Second, meat also contains considerable amounts of phosphorus and sulphur, minerals that are acid forming. Weston Price, a dentist, inventor, and researcher, conducted a few remarkable experiments in the early 1900s. His studies showed that when dogs were fed all meat diets, the animals began to show signs of osteoporosis, or thinning of the bones, because all the alkaline minerals like calcium, magnesium, manganese, zinc, and potassium, were used up to counterbalance the acids formed from the beef. This same process is the cause of bone and teeth demineralization in humans, as well as calcium depletion.

Did you know that Americans are the highest dairy consuming nation in the world, and yet we have the highest incidence of osteoporosis and incidences of broken bones and bone fractures? And what do we hear in commercials? "Got Milk?" We've all been brainwashed into believing that milk and dairy products put calcium in our bones when the opposite has been scientifically proven due to their body acidifying effects.

So what foods, lifestyle habits, or therapeutic methods are deacidifying, or have an alkalinizing effect? Again, fresh, raw, organic juicy fruits and vegetables have this effect. By juicy, I'm talking about those fruits and vegetables that have fairly high water contents such as cucumbers, carrots, melons, and green leafy vegetables—lettuces, chard, and kale.

Starchy fruits and vegetables such as bananas and potatoes are slightly acid forming. While it is important to have a balance of alkaline and acid-forming foods in your diet, the optimum diet would consist of 80% alkaline foods and 20% slightly acid forming foods. Despite this knowledge, most people eat much more acid-forming foods than their pH sensitive bodies can handle. Hence, our populations are afflicted with many modern plagues and chronic illnesses.

It is now widely recognized that an increase in alkalinizing foods will bring about a remarkable increase in energy, mental alertness, and better health in general. Earlier I mentioned that sports drinks that contain potassium can improve electrolyte balance, but, at the same time, may increase acidification and dehydration that can lead to joint and muscle spasms and pain. An athlete, running at top speed, will produce one-eighth ounce of lactic acid every second which amounts to half a pound in one minute. If this acid isn't neutralized, it accumulates and the runner becomes exhausted very quickly. To neutralize this acid, the athlete's blood needs to be as alkaline as possible. Therefore, drinking plenty of water and consuming more alkaline foods is the ticket to having the stamina needed to succeed in sports, or even be able to do a day of physical labor without getting tired and sore muscles from the buildup of lactic acid. Many people are suffering from chronic fatigue simply due to the accumulation of toxins caused from overconsumption of acid-forming foods and drink.

The more acidic your fluids and tissues become, the more subject they are to the growth of anaerobic bacteria, funguses, viruses, parasites, and various types of cancers. I have met a number of people who went through various detox programs, and alkalinized their bloodstream, to the point of having their parasites and certain cancers leave their bodies altogether. Remember, it's the acid wastes, and/or the accumulation of toxins in your body, that favor the growth of bacteria, cancer viruses, and causes increased susceptibility to infectious diseases due to immune suppression.

Finally, bioelectric therapies (discussed in detail in Chapter 6) may also help alkalinize your body. Relating this alkalinizing strategy to water, many people place magnets on their water pipes to help soften their drinking water. Similarly, this is a way to keep your shower doors and dishes spot free without installing an expensive water softener in your home. Place the north pole of the magnet, which tends to be alkalinizing, on the pipe. The south pole of a magnet is like the sun. It radiates outwardly and is stimulating. The north pole of a magnet in contrast is relaxing, like the moon, quieting or sedating.

This knowledge is put to use in cancer clinics, for example, in Mexico. Regular protocols include placing magnets directly on skin cancers intermittently for hours—an hour on and an hour off. This tends to make cancerous tumors more alkaline. Cancers, again, generally speaking, tend to grow in highly acidified terrains, approximately 4.0 to 5.0 pH.

According to a review article entitled "Diseased Cells and pH" in the scientific journal *Medical Hypothesis* (1994; 42:299-306), acidified serum surrounding cells not only slows normal cell division and growth, but also prompts premature aging. Scientific findings over the years prompted doctors Carlin and Carlin, from the Endocrinology Department of the Brooke Army Medical Center in San Antonio, Texas, to "wonder if aging was not, to a certain degree, just a slow progression of loss of ability to maintain a near alkaline state." Moreover, they advanced, substantial evidence showed that when cell growth mediums turn acidic, at least three mechanisms responsible for maintaining *intracellular* alkalinity are stressed. As a result, many cancer cells are prompted to grow due to the over compensation associated with pumping out excess acids out of viral infected, or genetically altered, cells. Thus, they concluded, abnormal *intracellular* alkalinity (in response to *extracellular* acidity) has a link to cancer, and this abnormal pH is considered essential for this disease to continue.

Finally, body acidity, poor circulation, and low oxygen levels go hand in hand. These co-factors all contribute to cancer as well as many other diseases. Cancers, for instance, typically grow in areas with poor circulation. Men get prostate cancers, and women get breast cancers in glands where blood flow is commonly restricted, oxygen levels fall, and acids build up. Colon cancers are linked likewise to over acidity wherein undigested foods ferment. This progressively creates more and more toxicity and acidity in the gut. As mentioned in the previous chapter, detoxification for these types of illnesses including colon cleansing strategies will help deacidify the colon.

Chapter 4.
Boosting Immunity

"I looked, and there before me was a pale horse!
Its rider was named Death,
and Hades was following close behind him.
They were given power over a fourth of the earth
to kill by sword, famine and plague, and by
the wild beasts of the earth."

Revelation 6:8,
The Holy Bible

As discussed on the audiotape programs *Horowitz "On Healing"* and *Preparing Your Temple of God: The End Times Sermon*, "step three" of my *Healing Celebrations* recommendations is boosting your immunity naturally. You have, thus far, learned how important it is to get rid of the toxic buildup in your body through various cleansing programs AND how important it is to deacidify your system through incorporating more alkaline foods and beverages as well as avoiding acidifying toxins such as caffeine, chocolate, nicotine, alcohol, prescription and nonprescription drugs, and refined carbohydrates, such as refined white sugar and white flour. This chapter directs your next step—boosting immunity. In other words, now that you have cleaned your "temple" and prepared it to receive God's Spirit, now, likewise, you can benefit by incorporating God's natural immune boosters in your life.

The Spirit of Natural Immunity

Very simply, God gave you a team of cells, tissues, and blood factors comprising the immune system to guard you against attack by foreign invading germs and toxins. Obviously, then, God wants you guarded and protected against disease and other evils.

Spiritually speaking, this immune system closely reflects your knowledge and appreciation of who you are as a whole human being, including your connection to God. Recent discoveries in the field of "psychoneuroimmunology"—the science dealing with the interrelationships between body, mind, emotions, behavior, and immunity, reveals an intimate association between spirituality and immunocompetence. Science is beginning to explain how positive emotions and attitudes like love, self-esteem, and meaningful purpose in life, empower natural immunity against various illnesses.

Thus, as a Holy child of God, you should be appreciative of your magnificence, how much God loves you, and your Spiritual connection, sometimes called the Holy Spirit. Knowledge of this fundamental connection between your spiritual "self" and your physical health contributes to complete self-knowledge, self-appreciation, self-esteem, and non-narcissistic self-love. These factors actually empower your immune system.

On the other hand, if you don't know or appreciate the magnificent person you are, and the miraculous healing powers that you hold, how can you expect your immune system to function optimally? Your immune system simply can't because its primary function is to differentiate "self" from "nonself." So if you don't know who you are, then your immune system will simply do likewise, unable to distinguish between your perfectly healthy cells and foreign invaders including cancers.

Most importantly, for health and longevity, you need to be Spiritually inspired while expressing your unique purpose in life.

My grandfather, Moses, was an excellent example of this. He stayed vitally alive for at least twenty years even though his bones and muscles were riddled with cancer. Thanks largely to medical doctors who promoted cigarette smoking when my grandfather was young, he became a chain smoker for more than seventy years. He developed cancer, but that wasn't what killed him.

My grandfather loved life for two reasons: number one was God, and number two was my grandmother, Betty. Moses consistently expressed his devotion through prayer and meditation which he did morning, noon, and night for three hours a day. The rest of his time he spent loving his wonderful wife. Caring for Betty was his Divine purpose in life. He shared everything he could with her. He died at age 93 when that purpose, to serve Betty, was denied him. My father and his brother committed Betty to a nursing home. Moses died three weeks later of a terminated life purpose and broken heart.

Moses's doctors couldn't figure out what killed him so quickly, so they ordered an autopsy. I was there when the surgeon came up from the morgue. He walked over to my father and said, "Mr. Horowitz, for the life of me, I can't understand how your dad could have lived for the past twenty years. Every single bone, muscle, and organ throughout his entire body was riddled with cancer."

My grandfather's story reflects the tremendous power that a spiritually inspired immune system has to maintain health and longevity. Like my grandfather, and everyone else, you have cancer cells growing in your body virtually all the time. The average person has 500 cancer cells growing at any moment. It is your immune system—your white blood cell "body guards" that seek and destroy those foreign invaders. A competent immune system, within a Spiritually inspired body, loves, nurtures, and supports that which is natural, healthy, and normal—cells given to you by God through His grace.

A Grave Challenge

Sadly, this is the major reason why the supreme focus of medical science for the past century has been on the immune system. Scientists and government officials proclaimed they were doing this research to stop immune rejections of grafts and organ transplants. But insidiously in the background, evil forces conspired to corrupt this most precious, God-given gift—the immune system—that functions as a virtual metaphor for self-esteem and God's love.

Military-medical-pharmaceutical industrialists recognized, early in the twentieth century, the critical role the immune system plays in protecting God's human treasures. In efforts to develop immune system destroying agents, including viruses and other infectious agents for germ warfare and population control, the military contractors that I exposed in *Emerging Viruses: AIDS & Ebola—Nature, Accident or Intentional?* (Tetrahedron, 1997) and *Healing Codes for the Biological Apocalypse* (Tetrahedron, 1999)—succeeded. Today, underlying every modern plague is grossly undermined "herd immunity." Agents for the Adversary of death and destruction labored to perfect ways to turn God's magnificent self-loving and nurturing system into a self-destroying autoimmune disease ravaging system. Today, industrialists make vast fortunes from humanity's suffering by doing just that—turning God's creations against themselves.

As I'll share in greater detail later, contaminated blood supplies and tainted vaccines have been primarily responsible for transmitting these immune system destroying agents, and conducting what amounts to global genocide. The entire array of autoimmune disorders have been generated this way. It is largely because of these evil efforts that cancer rates have skyrocketed during the past half century to today when half of the American people are expected to be diagnosed with cancer in their lifetimes.

Healing in a New Age of Fundamentalism

It's critical to boost your immune system every way possible—physically, mentally, emotionally, socially, environmentally, *and above all spiritually*—at this unique time in history. This is God's way of protecting your health and celebrating miraculous healings.

I emphasize spiritual blessings and healing herein because, again, it is most important. To build a stronger immune system, you need to create strong, vibrant, healthy cell structures and tissues that are filled with God's Holy Spirit and vibrate at a higher frequency of energy.

Many think the concept of healing through energy, sound, light, and special frequencies is "New Age." Later in this book I am going to discuss subjects that have been, in recent decades, vilified as too "New Age" for fundamentalist Christians. However, in light of recent Bible revelations published in the book *Healing Codes for the Biological Apocalypse*, and their implications and relationships to quantum physics, Pythagorean mathematics, and electromedicine, Christian fundamentalists, and everyone for that matter, should pray on this knowledge with heightened discernment. Whether you can appreciate it or not, as will be discussed in greater measure later, God's technologies for healing include the use of sound and crystals. His words are sound frequencies. They are electromagnetic mathematical expressions. His Divine light is likewise, as it flows freely and harmoniously through the Lord's instruments of love. Even crystals are used by God to transmit His healing vibrations, like those associated with the healing waters that Revelation predicts will flow through the "rivers and streams" of people who march triumphantly into the "Messianic New Age" of peace and prosperity. More revelations on these matters will follow later in this book.

Immune Boosting Supplements

During the past few decades there have been tremendous advances occurring in the fields of nutrition, biochemistry, and dietary supplementation. Modern healthcare has been virtually revolutionized by new knowledge and applications of natural vitamins, minerals, enzymes, herbs and plant extracts—also called "botanicals" and "phytonutrients." How can this knowledge affect you? What kinds of supplements should you be taking to achieve optimal vibrant health?

Green Harvest^{TM} is a good example of what I recommend, and take myself—a good tasting, smooth textured, powdered, whole food supplement. *Green Harvest*^{TM} contains minimally processed organically grown amaranth, brown rice, flaxseed, wheat grass, spirulina, millet, and much, much more. These whole foods, when blended together with juice and/or water, provide a highly nutritious and delicious immune booster formulated to produce results you should feel within a week.

Again, your best source of nutrients comes ideally from fresh organic foods. Thus, every morning I blend one scoop of *Green Harvest*^{TM}, a cup of good water, a cup of organic fruit juice, and a half banana per serving, to make a fruit smoothie for every member of my family. My children love it, and I can rest assured knowing they start each day with a good meal. They rarely get sick, even when exposed to cold and flu viruses in school. In the rare instance they do get sick, they quickly mount a solid immune response, and overcome the illness very fast compared to other children their ages.

With *Green Harvest*^{TM} you're not dealing with pharmaceutical-grade synthetic vitamins, like those found in most supplements purchased in drug stores. The famous name brand multivitamin tablets are typically bound with di-calcium phosphate, a binder that inhibits mineral absorption among other things.

In general, avoid all products that come in tablet form. Many brands from even bonafide "health food stores" contain this binder which renders their vitamins virtually useless, and actually inhibits the production of hydrochloric acid needed for digestion. This not only leaves you unable to assimilate the synthetic vitamins bound together by the di-calcium phosphate, but less able to effectively digest the foods you're eating as well.

Coffee, by the way, whether it is decaf or not, has a similar effect as di-calcium phosphate.

For most people, weeding through the myriad supplements available on the market today, without a degree in nutrition or herbology, can be an insurmountable task. I want to help you be able to distinguish the facts from fiction in today's world of mixed messages and downright propaganda.

An Interview with James South

James South is one of America's leading nutritional supplement formulators. He is extremely gifted in communicating technical information in easy to understand ways about how supplements work in your body.

In 1998, I had the opportunity to interview James for a three hour audiotape package entitled, *Nutritional Supplements for Immunity, Energy, Acuity, Rest and Recovery*. Here are some excerpts from his discussion on immune boosting supplements, and how you can benefit by taking them:

"There are many factors in your modern life that actually diminish the function of your immune system. Ironically, one of them is of course vaccinations, allegedly designed to enhance immune function, but when you look into the scientific research you find that it actually tends to pervert immune function in strange directions. It's no coincidence, for instance, that asthma and allergies have reached epidemic proportions in the late twentieth century, and so have autoimmune diseases where the human immune system, instead of attacking foreign germ invaders, attacks its own tissues, as in rheumatoid arthritis where it's attacking the joint tissues. What has happened is, vaccinations have caused our immune systems to become hyperactive—too active—in certain ways; ironically, often against their own tissues, or against harmless foreign invaders such as dust, pollens, or proteins from certain foods. At the same time, our immune systems have often become hypoactive—too little active—against the many bacterial, viral, fungal, and protozoal germ invaders that now, if anything, are more prevalent than they've been in a hundred years.

"So, part of what you need to do with your immune system is not strengthen it, but normalize it—to get it back on track. So that it leaves alone that which should be left alone—things like harmless dust mites, or your own tissues—and instead attacks the things that truly represent threats to the human body.

"You have to remember that the basic function of the immune system is to discriminate 'self' from 'nonself.' And when that 'nonself' is a harmful germ invader, to kill it fast before it can harm you.

"Additionally ironic, one of the boons of the twentieth century, especially if you live in a cold dry climate, is central indoor heating. This sets up the need for certain nutrients, just by the fact that you likely set your indoor Winter thermometer at 70 to 80 degrees Fahrenheit. But the first line of immune defense in the human body is the type of cells that line your nose, throat, sinuses, lungs, and entire intestinal tract. These are called mucous epithelial cells.

"When they're healthy, these mucous cells secrete enzymes called lysozymes. These lysozymes have the specific job of literally digesting, and thus destroying, any germs, be they bacteria, viruses or fungi, that might land on your nose, throat, or lung tissue from what you might breathe, drink, or inhale.

"Unfortunately, these mucous lining cells . . . can dry out, and then no longer perform their lysozyme secreting function.

"In addition, if the epithelial cells get too dried out, for too long, they actually change state. They do what is technically called 'keratinize.' That means they dry out, shrivel up, and may die. Then they can become food for the very bacteria that they were intended to kill.

Vitamin A

"Now it turns out that a specific vitamin has one of the major roles in maintaining the health of our epithelial cells. This vitamin is a rather humble vitamin, known for about a century, that people have largely forgotten. That is vitamin A. Vitamin A is a fat soluble vitamin. You can get it preformed from your diet if you happen to eat fish livers, which not many people do. Most of us get it in an alternative plant-based form called beta carotene, which, strictly speaking, isn't really vitamin A, but a healthy body can convert it into vitamin A in the liver as needed. When you have adequate vitamin A, this will go a long way towards making your epithelial cells resistant to that indoor heating, drying out, and damage that takes away your first line of immune defense.

"So vitamin A is one of the most important, yet overlooked, immune vitamins. In fact, in the 1940s and 1950s, in nutritional texts, it was often called the 'immune vitamin.'

"Most Americans don't get any preformed vitamin A. They get their vitamin A from their vegetables if they eat such in the form of beta-carotene. Unfortunately, science has discovered that there are many causes why some people may not successfully convert their beta-carotene into real vitamin A.

"For example, high levels of nitrates and nitrites, which are common fertilizers that have leached into water supplies, [and also commonly found in processed preserved deli meats] will impair beta-carotene conversion to vitamin A."

Other risks undermining the conversion of beta carotene to vitamin A, James relayed, include: insulin deficiencies, high stress, and steroid exposures including natural corticosteroid release, and man-made prednisone.

"An ingredient that I believe is most beneficial to an immune supplement," James continued, "are preformed vitamin A, called retinyl-palmitate, at a significant, but nontoxic, level. [Approximately 6,000 international units (I.U.) will do for this.] As well as an even larger amount of beta carotene [9,000 I.U.]. The nice thing about beta carotene is the body will not convert it if there is more than enough vitamin A. So there's no potential toxicity with beta carotene. . . . In fact, your liver can store a five year supply of vitamin A with no problem.

"Now you may have heard that vitamin A is a potentially toxic vitamin. It's one of the few nutrients that has any, even remote, possibility of significant toxicity associated with it. In the real world, however, vitamin A toxicity is much more of a myth than a reality. Among adult human beings it's extremely unusual to develop even mild cases of vitamin A toxicity, which is a completely reversible problem, anyway, at doses less than 50,000 I.U. per day for a long period of time. I have taken, for instance, 25,000 units to 100,000 units of vitamin A each day continuously for twenty-six years, and I'm still here to tell you about it. So vitamin A, yes it can be toxic, but in the real world you have to work at it, if you are an adult. . . . Children under five, however, you especially need to be more careful with vitamin A. They are a lot more sensitive on a pound-for-pound bodyweight basis than adults. . . .

More Problems For Immunity With Vaccines

"Now another problem with vaccinations is that when they introduce these possibly killed germs, or germ proteins, into your bloodstream, they bypass the normal mucous barriers of your body by direct injection through the skin.

"A great thing about mucous tissues, whether you're talking the intestinal lining, or the lungs, . . . is that a certain type of white blood cell hangs out there just waiting for germs to make it through your first line of defense. This type of white blood cell is called a *macrophage*. The word derives from the Greek words meaning 'big eaters.' They are like the garbage disposal units of the immune system. They have a wide ranging diet. They'll eat almost anything that shouldn't be in your body—even little particles of carbon, as well as germs and foreign proteins. They're not picky; they eat it all. Yet these macrophages are lodged in with your mucous tissues. That, again, is your first line of immune defense—not only the mucous lysozymes, but also the 'big eaters.'

"When macrophages attack germs they literally engulf them. They surround them with their protoplasm—their tissue. The germs go inside the macrophages which then secrete enzymes which kill and break germs down into fragments.

"Now the macrophage's job doesn't stop here. In many ways the macrophage is the Paul Revere of the immune system. It sends out the alarm if too many germs are coming in, and the macrophage begins to realize your body is under germ attack. It sends out immune signals, like Paul Revere riding through the streets of Boston saying, 'The red germs are coming! The red germs are coming!'

"So when you bypass the epithelial tissues which harbor these macrophages, [by needle injections of vaccines] you bypass this first link in the up-regulation of the immune system from a standby status into an active attack status.

"Another function your macrophages have is to take little bits of the dead germs that they've broken down, and then present them to another type of immune cell called the *B-cells*, or B-type white blood cell lymphocytes. This transfer of information acts like a computer program telling these B-lymphocytes what kind of specific antibodies to make to fight these incoming germs.

"Antibodies are like guided missiles that have the name of a specific germ on them. There may be, for example, a 'measles antibody,' or an 'anthrax antibody.' And your body can't be wasting its resources making antibodies against every single germ on earth. Rather, your body waits to up-regulate production of more antibodies against a specific germ when it gets the message that this specific germ has invaded.

"So your macrophages play a critical role in transferring the specific information to your B-cells required for an adequate antibody response against the specific invader.

"This is one of the many dark sides of vaccination," James concluded. "It simply bypasses, and in some ways dis-regulates," this normal immune system programming method.

Vaccines and Autoimmune Diseases

Another way in which your immune system gets fooled and undermined by vaccinations involves the formation of "antigenic complexes." An antigenic complex forms when a foreign protein combines with your own body protein. That is, when you get vaccinated, bits and pieces of bacteria, viruses, fungi, and other species of animal proteins get injected into your bloodstream. These particles, mostly proteins, attach themselves to your own cellular proteins. This forms a "complex." Your body now recognizes this entire complex as *foreign*, and mounts an "autoimmune" attack against the entire complex. Your own body begins to destroy itself—that is, antigenic complexes which include your own cells and tissues get attacked by antibodies and macrophages. This best explains a host of autoimmune diseases including: chronic fatigue immune dysfunction (CFIDS), fibromyalgia, lupus, multiple sclerosis, rheumatoid arthritis, type 1 diabetes, and many, many others.

Zinc—The Immune System Mineral

"Just as vitamin A is 'the immune vitamin,' the trace mineral zinc is 'the immune mineral," James South continued. "Zinc has multiple functions in enhancing and potentiating your immune system.

"One of the many things that zinc does is it escorts vitamin A out of the liver. You can take and store up all of the vitamin A you want, . . . but if you're deficient in zinc, you'll have problems getting the vitamin A out of the liver and into your bloodstream.

"Zinc and vitamin A together combine with a certain type of protein in the liver called albumin. And then they travel throughout the bloodstream to deliver the vitamin and zinc to wherever they are needed. So one of zinc's first immune functions is, simply, to get vitamin A where it needs to go to perform its immune functions.

"Although the recommended daily allowance, the RDA, of zinc has been set at 15 milligrams (mgs.) per day by the government, there is a lot of evidence that probably more like 20, 30 or even 40 mgs. is a more realistic dosage for immune competence and optimal health. Even by RDA standards, typical dietary surveys show the average American gets somewhere between 7 and 11 mgs. of zinc per day. So typically you may only be getting between a half or two-thirds of the RDA anyway. So zinc isn't exactly plentiful in your average diet. Especially if you eat a junk food, or refined food, diet.

"In addition, certain fibers in diets, including wheat bran fiber that many elderly people take as an inexpensive dietary source of fiber to combat constipation, ironically, is a very good complexer with zinc. It renders zinc nonabsorbable, so it sends your zinc right down the toilet. . . . So zinc is something that people are typically inadequately supplied with."

"Zinc and vitamin A are also needed to strengthen and protect the brain of your immune system, which is a little gland in your chest called the thymus gland. This tiny thymus gland that weighs less than an ounce, roughly behind where your 'V-notch'—is on your breast bone, is a multi-pronged computer, director, and energizer for your immune forces. One of its functions is to secrete various immune hormones with names like thymosin, thymopentin, and thymopoietin which are the signaling devices that direct the different branches of your immune system—much like the Army, Navy, Air Force, and Marines. These are coordinated and directed by these immuno-hormones from the thymus gland. This makes the gland very important. But that's not all that it does!

"When white blood cells are immature, they must be put through 'boot camp' so to speak, and turned into immune fighter killer warriors. This 'boot camp' literally occurs in the thymus gland. Immature white blood cell body guards are programmed in the thymus gland, and actually changed in their structure and function therein, to exit the gland being killer white blood cells at war with foreign invaders. At this point they are called T-lymphocytes. The 'T' stands for thymus.

"Ironically, the thymus gland is easily damaged and shriveled-up by our own stress hormone cortisol. Cortisol is such a powerful immune suppressor, in part by shriveling-up the thymus gland, that if you were to have an organ transplant, your doctor would put you permanently on immune suppressive drugs so that your body would not reject the foreign organ. In that case, it might be a necessary evil—the best you can hope for. But the doctors would likely give you a synthetic form of cortisol, simulating your own stress hormone called prednisone, to suppress your immune system.

"Well, your own naturally secreted cortisol, when you're stewing in your own stress juices for long periods of time, will also shrivel up and shrink your own thymus gland. This is called thymus involution. One of the ironies is that by the time you are a teenager, your thymus gland is typically a fraction of the size that was when you were a healthy ten-year-old. Already the stress of life has taken its toll."

Reflecting on medical history for a moment, in the 1950s, American doctors would occasionally find a teenager with a large thymus gland. They often thought it was abnormal, much like a tumor, since they rarely saw that kind of thing. In the 1950s, the rage became burning out the "excess" thymus gland tissue with x-ray radiation. What was ultimately proven was that these teens had actually been among the fortunate few whose thymus had been spared the stress of life! This unfortunate piece of medical history is similar to the simultaneous surgical stampede to remove children's tonsils to relieve periodic "strep throats." Again, it was later determined that this practice was not only unnecessary, but actually harmful. It compromised natural immunity against all types of infections, including "strep throat!"

In summary, the trace mineral zinc, along with vitamin A, can prevent what is called thymus involution or thymus shrinkage. They keep the thymus in a healthy, active/functional state so you can keep your immune warriors armed for battle and in communication with operations central.

Free Radicals and Zinc

Finally, zinc is also part of a very important antioxidant complex called zinc-SOD. This plays a role in neutralizing the dangerous reactive free radicals that increase your risk for getting cancers. Free radicals were discussed briefly in the previous chapter regarding ionization and acid/base balance. Free radicals are tiny electron particles that can spin off from atoms and molecules in your body and can damage cells and tissues. Free radicals form, for example, during exposures to x-ray radiation from every source—natural background, nuclear, or medical radiation. The build up of these free radicals is what causes death following excessive radiation exposures. The free radicals break down human tissue so dramatically that following exposure to a massive burst of radiation, the free radicals formed might actually melt the flesh off of your bones within hours. The free radicals then literally dissolve all the cellular structures of your body.

Yet, free radicals, according to James South, are a dual edged sword. A certain modest amount of them are actually needed for health. Specifically, the way that your immune cells destroy invading germs is by first surrounding the microbes, and then barraging them with certain types of free radicals. One is called myeloperoxidase. Another is called hydroxyl free radicals; another is hydrogen peroxide, and another, superoxide. "A host of different free radicals are used like artillery by your white blood cell body guards to destroy invading germs.

"When immune cells secrete free radicals, some of these leak out into your bloodstream. This is one of the causes of general malaise—feeling rotten, pained, toxic, and fatigued—when you get really sick. You may feel like there's a war going on inside of you, and that's precisely what is happening in-so-far-as the immune system is concerned.

"An important factor that helps to minimize the destruction associated with this battle for health freedoms within you is antioxidant enzymes and antioxidant nutrients. Antioxidants are nature's neutralizers of free radicals. They literally combine with free radicals and neutralize them like water putting out a fire.

"One of the great things about zinc is that your body uses it to make one of the main antioxidant enzymes—zinc-SOD. This stands for zinc superoxide dismutase. The more of these antioxidant enzymes and nutrients you have, the more your body cannot be bothered by the inevitable free radical leakage from your white blood cells."

Vitamin C

There is a massive amount of scientific evidence that shows vitamin C plays a variety of roles in either aiding your immune system, or acting as a molecular parallel immune system. Thus, to say that vitamin C can't help in fighting colds or worse infections is simply *hogwash*!

For example, James South relayed a 1978 study by two Japanese scientists—Murashege and Murata. They published their results of giving intravenous vitamin C to about 1500 patients who had to receive blood transfusions in Japanese hospitals. One of the risks of receiving transfused blood is hepatitis, which can be associated with either bacterial or viral agents. During this double blind study, the scientists gave about 190 people a placebo—a harmless inert substance, and another 1500 people vitamin C in multigram dosages intravenously—directly into their bloodstreams. They found that of those who received the placebo, no vitamin C, they developed thirteen cases of hepatitis. That equated to a seven percent infection rate. Among the 1500 people that got vitamin C, there was only five cases. That equaled a three-tenths of one percent infection rate—a strikingly significant risk reduction! That is, the vitamin C group had less than 1/20th the hepatitis rate under similar transfusion conditions.

So one of the things that is proven about vitamin C, is that when the levels are high enough in your bloodstream, vitamin C will combine with *oxygen* (which will be discussed in greater detail in the following chapter), and generate a type of free radical called the ascorbyl-free radical, which will directly kill the germs independent of your immune system having to lift a finger on its own. So in a sense, *vitamin C is an independent molecular immune system.*

Therefore, when you maintain high blood levels of vitamin C—from 6,000 to 20,000 milligrams throughout the day—as many health conscious people do, this can profoundly increase your immunity against infectious microbes, especially deadly viruses, through this ascorbyl-free radical mechanism.

Other known functions of vitamin C include enhanced antibody production and response to infectious agents; protection against the ravaging effects of cortisol and subsequent thymus gland destruction, anti-aging, and much more.

Given the above knowledge, one of the best forms of vitamin C that you can take to enhance immune functions is zinc ascorbate—vitamin C linked to the immune mineral zinc.

Other Immune-Related Trace Minerals

The trace mineral iodine, combined with potassium to form potassium iodide, can enhance the immune system through the production, by white blood cells, of an enzyme called myeloperoxidase. The core of this enzyme contains the iodine atom. Thus, if you lack sufficient iodine in your diet, you're at risk for reduced immunity through insufficient myeloperoxidase production.

As mentioned in chapter 3, many people are becoming wise to the risks of consuming iodized salt, or standard table salt, for their source of iodine. Too much table salt, you learned, can cause acid/base chemistry imbalances, fluid retention, as well as hypertension or high blood pressure.

However, there are many regions of the country where environmental iodine is lacking. These have been called the "goiter regions," that include the "goiter belt"—the American Midwest—due to the development of hyperthyroidism related to the reduction of available iodine. For this reason, the RDA level of iodine for your diet, or found in a good supplement in the form of potassium iodide, is 150 micrograms.

Other trace minerals that should be included in well formulated nutritional supplements include at least: 1 mg. of copper, 90 mg. of magnesium, and 160 mcg. of selenium.

Other Unique Immune Boosters

During the last part of the twentieth century, a host of unique substances were isolated, tested, and found to help promote immunocompetence. These include: coenzyme Q_{10}, N-acetyl cysteine, cat's claw, astragalus extract, turmeric extract, green tea extract, propolis extract, and olive leaf extract.

Coenzyme Q_{10} is a very expensive nutrient that your body can theoretically make, but not always make enough. Evidence shows that with aging, less and less CoQ_{10} is produced so that by old age your risk of developing congestive heart failure increases significantly. CoQ_{10} has also been shown to relay important immune boosting functions. The minimum useful dose of CoQ_{10} found in good human supplements is 30 mg.

Plant derived nutrients, called "phytonutrients" found to have immune boosting effects include a Chinese tonic herb known as astragalus. A seventy percent concentrate, 300 mg. dose, of this herb contains polysaccharides, related to complex sugars, proven by the Chinese to stimulate macrophages to become more vigilant and active. Astragalus is, therefore, a specific vitamin tonic for the macrophages of your body. This, again, helps your first line of immune defense.

Cat's claw extract, also known as Una de Gato, is a Peruvian herb that contains an exotic class of chemicals called indole-alkaloids. These alkaloids have also been shown to activate antibody production, and the release of immune hormones called cytokines and lymphokines. 100 mg. of this extract is often found in well formulated supplements.

From Asia comes one of the most ancient, treasured, and simple, remedies called green tea. Studies of people living in rural Japan, who lived to a ripe old age, found that they drank five or more cups of green tea daily. They also had significantly less cancers, tooth decay, and had healthier immune systems. The active chemicals in green tea are called polyphenols. 200 mg. of a 52% extract of green tea provides the equivalent of drinking five strong cups.

Propolis concentrate is a salivary secretion from honey bees, or better known in the industry as "bee spit." It is the substance that bees plaster all over their hives. The reason they do this is because propolis is a direct broad spectrum germicide. It keeps their beehives free from infectious germs and the bee colony healthy. Propolis concentrate has been used for ages. Beekeepers commonly eat propolis along with raw honeycomb honey and, as a result, live to ripe old ages and have very sound immune systems. A 250 mg. dose of propolis extract might therefore be found in a good supplement.

Finally, two sulphur amino acids that play key roles in immune health include N-acetyl cysteine and taurine. These nutrients are used by the body to make a very important substance called glutathione. This is a simple molecule composed of three protein building blocks—amino acids, that play an important role inside cells of immune compromised people such as HIV/AIDS patients. Glutathione is made from the sulphur amino acid cysteine, but, unfortunately, when we get cysteine either in food or a supplement, 80% of the important side of the molecule—the sulph-hydryl group, breaks off due to your stomach acid. Then the molecule does little good in the production of glutathione. But N-acetyl cysteine is a superior form of cysteine, wherein the acetyl group—like the acid in vinegar—acts like a shield to save the sulph-hydryl so that you only lose about 20% of the molecule during digestion and absorption. N-acetyl cysteine in human and animal tests has been shown to induce, or increase, this all important glutathione.

Glutathione is also very important in relation to your antioxidant response to free radicals. There are many different antioxidants in your body. One is vitamin C. Others include vitamin E, zinc, selenium, beta-carotene, and lipoic acid. Each of these sacrifice themselves when they destroy free radicals, but then these become what they destroyed—free radicals. With glutathione available, these vitamins and nutrients get recycled.

Glutathione is also the raw material for one of the most important antioxidant enzymes called glutathione peroxidase. This is also required to mop up the hydrogen peroxide that virtually every white blood cell leaks as it destroys invading germs. This hydrogen peroxide could harm your own tissues if not checked by glutathione peroxidase.

Also, another component of glutathione peroxidase is the trace mineral selenium. Very few Americans get adequate selenium in their diets because the soils have been dramatically depleted of it. Some of it is still found in the "heartland" of the Midwest and the Rocky Mountains.

Minimal amounts of N-acetyl cysteine, and selenium, found in well formulated supplements are 400 mg. and 160 mcg. respectively.

A small amount of copper, 1 mg. daily, which is half of the RDA, acts as an essential trace mineral to play an important role in immune system health. Too much copper may be toxic. It is one of the few minerals you need to be concerned about, insofar as too much may be harmful. This, as mentioned above, works with vitamin C to form the ascorbyl-free radical that helps defend against infectious germs.

Vitamin E

You may have heard that Vitamin E is critical for a healthy heart and cardiovascular system. 400 to 800 mg. of d-alpha tocopherol, natural vitamin E, per day is highly recommended for a healthy immune system. What is natural Vitamin E? There is a variety of E vitamins on the market—some natural and others synthetic. That's why it's imperative that you read the label before you purchase! Make sure you purchase *d-alpha tocopherol* or d-alpha tocopherol acetate. These forms are the most potent forms and the most bio-available. Mixed tocopherols simply means that the beta, gamma, and delta tocopherols are added in with the alpha tocopherol. There is very little known biological activity with any of these other tocopherols, which is why I recommend purchasing d-alpha tocopherol. The biggest problem with many of the vitamin E products on the market, particularly the vitamin E in standard multivitamins, is that they often use a cheap synthetic source of vitamin E. The label says "dl-alpha tocopherol." When you see the "l" after the d, don't buy it! If you have any at home, throw it away! This synthetic vitamin E is toxic. Do any of you remember the Cambridge diet? They used this synthetic Vitamin E—dl-alpha tocopherol, and many people developed headaches and soreness in their muscles as a result.

Additional Nutritional Notes

Generally speaking, the best supplements are the most bio-available. These will often contain one or more of the micro-algaes like spirulina, chlorella, and blue-green algaes.

Nutritional supplementation is one area in which it is not worth it to pinch pennies. After all, what can possibly be more important than your health and vitality, or the health of your family and loved ones? We are certainly living in challenging times, and I can't stress enough how important it is to become more discerning in the choices you make while you continually ask for your Creator's guidance.

Getting "Raped" By "Canola Oil"

I want to briefly cover the topic of oils, essential fatty acids, margarine versus butter, and the *dangers* of low fat, high protein diets commonly used today.

What kind of oils should you use? Olive oil, the first cold pressing, is by far the healthiest oil to use. Other oils that are beneficial are cold-pressed and unrefined sunflower, safflower, and sesame seed oils. These oils must be refrigerated. Any oil (or food) that has a long shelf life outside of the refrigerator has very little food value and is often, actually detrimental to your health.

If you've been led to believe that "canola oil," also called "rapeseed oil," is good for you, you've been had. Being a mono-saturated oil, like olive oil, one might think it's healthy. It has, after all, been promoted as a healthy and economical alternative to olive oil. Although, canola oil may be monosaturated, and economical, it is far from healthy. Canola is a coined word for rapeseed. You must admit that "canola" sounds better than "rape." The name actually disguised the introduction of "rape" oil to America.

Indeed, canola oil comes from the rape seed, which is part of the mustard family of plants. *Rape is the most toxic of all food-oil plants.* Both soy and rape are weeds. Insects won't eat either plant since they are both poisonous to them, but the *oil from the rape seed is one hundred times more toxic than soy oil!*

Canola, or rapeseed, is an industrial oil that is used as a lubricant, fuel, soap, a synthetic rubber base, and as an illuminant for the slick color pages you see in magazines. As an industrial oil, it does *not* belong in the human body! This oil has some very interesting characteristics and effects on living systems. For example, it forms latex-like substances that agglutinate red blood corpuscles. That means, the red cells stick together into lazy strands. Soy oil does the same thing to red cells, but not nearly as much.

Rape oil is also known to antagonize the central and peripheral nervous systems. Loss of vision is a known and common side-effect. Again, soy oil does the same, but far less. This deterioration often takes years and is associated with emphysema, respiratory distress, anemia, constipation, irritability, and blindness in animals and in humans.

Rape oil was widely used in animal feeds throughout England between 1986 and 1991, whereafter it was thrown out. Do you remember reading about the cows, pigs, and sheep that went blind, lost their minds, attacked people, and had to be shot? The experts blamed their disease on scrapie—a disease first thought to be linked to "slow viruses," and later to prion protein crystals. Their resulting brain holes caused the animals to behave erratically. But, when the rape seed oil was removed from their diets, their "scrapie" disappeared. Today, "scrapie-like" illness seems to be spreading rapidly throughout the world in humans in the form of Creutzfeldt-Jakob disease (CJD). It makes you wonder how much of this may be associated with brain damage from dietary canola, doesn't it?

Industry experts love to tell us how canola was developed in Canada and is safe to use. This is how the name canola was coined—CANadian OIL. They even admit that it was developed from rape seeds, through genetic engineering and irradiation, after which it is no longer rape seed but "canola" instead.

Over the past few decades U.S. and Canadian farmers have grown more and more rape seed for use by canola oil manufacturers. They ship it for use in thousands of processed foods, with the blessings of our governments, and watchdog agencies, particularly the powerful and corrupt FDA. I say "corrupt" for several reasons, the least of which is they "fast-track" for approval costly and toxic cancer and AIDS drugs, and condone distribution of toxic canola oil, while persecuting those dispensing virtually harmless vitamins and herbs.

Canola's Relative—Nerve Gas?

Rape oil is also the source of the infamous chemical-warfare agent, mustard gas, which was banned after blistering the lungs and skin of thousands of soldiers and civilians during World War I. Recent French reports indicate that it was again used during the Gulf War.

Canola oil contains large amounts of cyanide containing compounds called isothiocyanates. Its chemical relative, cyanide, inhibits mitochondrial production of your body's major energy molecule called ATP, short for adenosine triphosphate. This energy molecule fuels virtually every metabolic function.

Canola oil is also high in glycosides. Glycosides are best known as the component in rattlesnake venom that inhibits muscle enzymes and causes instant immobilization of the victim. By blocking certain enzyme functions, and depleting your

76

bioelectric energy, canola oil can actually interfere with critical biochemical processes in humans and animals.

Canola oil, as well as soy oil containing glycosides, can also depress your immune system. These oils can cause your white-blood-cell body guards, your T-cells, to go into a stupor and fall asleep on the job. So you can now see how the proliferation of these oils in the foods we eat can contribute to the increased risk of immune system deficiency disorders.

Fluoride, chloride, aspartame, vaccinations, malathion sprayed as an insecticide, ethylene dibromide in jet fuel and their "chemtrails," antibiotics, and junk foods all play a similar role in weakening immune systems.

Given this mix of toxic liabilities, the least you can do to limit your exposures is to check the ingredients in your processed foods. Most mayonnaise, for example, is made with soy or canola oils. Even some "health food stores" promote canola oil as preferable to other oils. If you look at many commercial brand peanut butters, you'll notice that they've replaced the peanut oil with canola oil.

Essential and Nonessential Fats

Moving ahead on the topic of which fats are truly healthy and which ones are downright dangerous. The questions you want to ask are: 1) How natural is this product? 2) How much is this product processed? 3) Will animals eat it? 4) Will it keep well outside my refrigerator? In other words, is the shelf life so long as to render the product dead and totally devoid of any nutritional value?

When it comes to butter versus margarine, the answer is pretty clear that butter is the preferred choice. Try feeding margarine to your dog or cat. They won't eat it. The reason is because margarine is horrible for your health. It is composed of artificially hydrogenated oils. It is the hydrogenation of oils, and the homogenization of milk, that can interfere with your body's ability to produce natural "good" cholesterol, among other things.

Many people blame saturated fats from meats and dairy products on the current epidemic of cardiovascular diseases, when the problem is actually refined hydrogenated fats and oils. Many people do themselves more harm than good with low-fat diets. Your immune, digestive, cardiovascular, and neurological systems, as well as your skin, are dependent on essential fatty acids.

Essential fatty acids are structural components of cell membranes, and precursors to the prostaglandin hormones needed for normal immune function. Prostaglandins also control many metabolic processes. These polyunsaturated fats are called "essential" because your body can't manufacture them. They must come from your diet. Having a deficit of essential fatty acids in modern diets can be a major contributing factor in the current epidemics of allergies and neurological diseases.

You need a healthy amount of fat in your diet, but the amount and type of fat eaten determines how it is used. There's a crucial difference between structural and storage fat. Structural fat is a major component of cell membranes, internal organs, and brain and nervous tissue (the myelin that "sheaths" your nerves is 79% fat!!) Essential fatty acids are a vital part of structural fat, so that when your diet is lacking in the healthy essential fatty acids, the deficiency impacts the functioning of your nervous system in a major way.

Storage fat, on the other hand, is fat used by your body as a "food reserve." Today, with refrigerators and supermarkets storing food, you don't need much fat to function likewise. Yet, most Americans continue to accumulate it! Obesity, or storage fat, has become excessive in developed nations as a direct result of eating a diet rich in processed foods, loaded with sugar, refined grains, animal fat, as well as hydrogenated and high-temperature processed vegetable oils. Even the livestock we eat has been turned obese through chemical and hormonal manipulation.

Junk food diets are so nutrient-poor that they require an over-consumption of calories to compensate. You end up depleting your body's nutrient stores every time you eat junk, including that doughnut and cup of coffee you crave. You can't fool your body for long. When your body lacks essential fatty acids, and other nutrients, you will tend to go on eating binges until you satisfy your body's need for these nutrients.

There is a lot of propaganda centered around saturated fats being harmful. The people of Southeast Asia have eaten saturated fats in the forms of coconut and palm oils for centuries and still maintain a low prevalence of heart disease. The Eskimos have also eaten excessive amounts of whale blubber, and other fatty meats, as part of their traditional diet, and they don't experience the cardiovascular problems that most North Americans do. In fact, human breast milk—the most natural of human foods—is around 45% saturated fat!

One side note, baby formulas are often soy based and nearly devoid of essential fatty acids. Based on clinical observations, it appears that sudden infant death (SIDS), and other vaccine related injuries, may be substantially reduced by breast-feeding if the mother eats a healthy diet rich in essential fatty acids.

What is the best source of essential fatty acids? Whole grains, nuts, seeds and, my favorite, avocados. Even health food stores are now carrying flax seed oils, and other high quality oils, that have a higher percentage of these beneficial fatty acids.

Garlic As An Antibiotic

Garlic is a fabulous antibiotic. Parents who run to their physicians with children who have ear infections, can save themselves, and their kids, a lot of grief.

Again, one of the most common vaccine related injuries are the chronic ear infections that are now epidemic in our children. Why? Because when you vaccinate, you actually *weaken* your entire immune system.

My children, for instance, who have never been vaccinated, sometimes swim in contaminated waters. Both of our girls swim like fish, so we can't keep them out of the ocean, pools, lakes, and swimming holes. Thus, occasionally, they may get ear infections due to unexpected contaminations. Rather than rush to see the pediatrician, I take a clove of garlic, mince it up, and drop some distilled water into the minced up garlic. Then I take a Q-tip and moisten it with the "garlic juice." I put them to bed on their sides with their infected ears facing up. Then I just touch the damp Q-tip onto the skin of the outer ear canals. If they were awake it might sting a little, but by the next morning their earaches are gone.

We've used this garlic remedy time and time again. It has always worked. That's not to say that cases of severe inner ear infections, and other causes of earaches, for example, neurological, don't require professional diagnosis and treatment. But, in most cases of outer ear infections, garlic earns its name as "the Russian penicillin."

When a terrible flu hit Russia at the turn of the century, people there discovered that consuming large quantities of garlic minimized their symptoms. Many averted the disease altogether. The value of garlic as a powerful immune system stimulant was finally recognized, at least among the Russian peasants and the international alternative health community that caught wind of it.

A popular garlic-based anti-plague remedy that Dr. Richard Schultz recommends, that will keep your immune system strong so that you don't catch every cold or flu that's going around, is easily made as follows: Buy three quarters of a pound of each of the following: organic garlic, organic white onion, horseradish root, ginger root, and the hottest habanero peppers you can find. Put these five ingredients, finely chopped, into a widemouth gallon glass jar and fill the jar up the rest of the way with raw, organic apple cider vinegar from your health food store. Shake the ingredients in the jar over the course of two weeks and then strain off some for daily use during the cold/flu season.

A friend recently told me that after a particularly stressful week at work, he felt a flu bug coming on. He was feeling chilled and ached all over, so he took 2-3 ounces of Dr. Schultz's concoction then went to bed. The next morning he was amazed. He felt wonderful.

You really don't need to run to your physician's office to get antibiotics every time you get sick. Especially since antibiotics typically acidify your body and weaken your immune system! The acidity and kill-off of resident microbes in your body creates even greater susceptibility to fungal infections. This is a major problem today, especially with the upper respiratory infections and flu-like illnesses going around. Be wise. The simple, tried and true, God-given, natural healing remedies are truly what are called for at this time.

Transfer Factors and Immunity

Among the highly effective, and largely suppressed, areas of alternative medicine are *transfer factors*. Transfer factors are powerful chemical messengers that relay immunity to infectious agents such as bacteria and viruses. Far safer than today's vaccines, but like vaccines, transfer factors work by alerting your immune cells that infectious microbes exist in the world, and that at some point your immune system might be called upon to fight them.

Transfer factors are far superior to vaccines in that they are free from bacteria, viruses, foreign RNA and DNA, animal proteins, and other typical vaccine ingredients including formaldehyde, formalin, MSG, mercury, and aluminum derivatives.

Years ago, research showed that, rather than vaccinate, you could accomplish virtually the same response, if not better immunity, without the unnecessary risk, by developing and isolating *transfer factors* from animals. Researchers began by infecting animals, for example, cows, with the germs against which they wished to immunize humans. They then isolated the T-type white blood cells from the infected cows—those immunological body guards that relayed the chemical messages needed to direct the immune response. Then they isolated the chemical messages themselves. Lo and behold, they now had the specific chemical message units responsible for directing a substantial immune response against a certain germ if and when it appeared. All immunity transferred orally, by way of a pill, without getting stuck with needles and injected with toxic particles!

In other words, the stimulated white blood cells produce a tiny chemical that alerts the entire immune system that it has seen a particular bacteria or virus, and to be prepared for a possible infection. These chemical message units were called "transfer factors." Today, and for years now, they've been able to isolate these transfer factors, and give them to people to "transfer" immunity against certain germs without using risky vaccines.

So if you want to raise your body's immunity against a particular microorganism, or help prevent or even help reverse some of the vaccine injuries, transfer factors may be helpful. Research is currently underway to produce a combination of transfer factors that incorporates all the risky childhood vaccinations without transferring the risks.

Other Immune Risks and Stress as a Co-Factor

So far I have written about the physical aspect of keeping your immune system in good shape. What about the mental, emotional, social, environmental, and above all the spiritual aspects of health? You've got to be concerned about those as well. Emotionally and mentally you want to reduce stress. Please understand that most of your stress is caused by communication breakdowns in your family or at work. You must learn how to communicate assertively and above all lovingly. This knowledge, and exercises to develop these skills, are thoroughly covered in my nine-hour audiotaped interactive training program called *Taking Care of Yourself.*

Again, you should take care of yourself every way possible, but if you don't have your relationship right with God you are *nowhere*! It is through your spiritual connection to God, and then your rapport with people, that you can best feel fulfilled and purposeful. Purpose in life is the fabric of society. Godly people all have a desire to share and care and love and help other people. To serve "thy neighbor as thyself" is the driving force inspiring life and social contribution.

It is the great Father in heaven who made and gave you everything, including your power. It's both humbling and empowering to know that you are a Holy child of God, connected to His incredible power. You have God's love and energy flowing through your immune system that you can put to work in your life to propel your vitality to fulfill your special purpose.

When you really know who you are, when you comprehend this sacred knowledge and special meaning in your life, it will become a vital part of your journey here on earth. As Yeshua's brother James wrote in the Bible (James 1:2), "the testing of your trust produces perseverance.... [S]o that you may be complete and whole, lacking in nothing." Later, I'll touch on Yeshua's council regarding lack of trust, resulting in stress and anger, violating your Divine empowerment including your capacity to produce miracles.

Again, if you respect and love the "complete and whole" person you are, only then can you expect your immune system to do likewise while keeping your microbial enemies away. Trusting this gift to respond successfully to "tests" and stress, as God planned it, will profoundly enhance your health, happiness, and longevity.

Chapter 5.
Oxygenation Therapies
and Related Godly Practices

"Then, God formed a person
from the dust of the ground
and breathed into his nostrils the breath of life,
so that he became a living being. . . ."
Receive meekly the word implanted in you
that can save your lives."

Genesis 2:7 and James 1:2,
The Holy Bible

Now for the fun part of the *Healing Celebrations* prescription—oxygenation and bioelectric technologies. For reasons that will become obvious to you in this chapter, these two overlapping forms of natural healing have been heavily suppressed, and those teaching and practicing them persecuted.

First, what is oxygen? The earth is composed of over 100 elements and among the most abundant of all of them is oxygen. In its simplest form, oxygen is a single atom symbolized by the letter "O" (sometimes referred to as "singlet oxygen"). The most well known and most common form of oxygen is when two atoms combine to make molecular oxygen known as "O_2." Ozone is a larger more reactive form of oxygen that contains three atoms of oxygen, and is symbolized by "O_3."

Where does oxygen come from? Mostly photosynthesis. Green trees produce it continuously. We mostly think of oxygen in the air we breathe, but, in fact, it is everywhere. All living matter contains oxygen. Besides breathing it, you drink it and consume it in your foods. It is naturally found in combination with other elements in water, in all organic compounds such as carbohydrates (sugars, starches, cellulose, fiber), glycogenic fats, and proteins. Even the clay and rock structures of soils are loaded with oxygen containing compounds in the form of oxides, hydroxides, carbonates, sulfates, and others.

How important is it? There is no other substance on which we are so dependent. We can go for weeks without food and days without water, but we can't go for minutes without oxygen. Probably the most recognized result of decreased oxygen in your body is a lack of energy. On the other hand, increased energy levels commonly occur with higher oxygen levels in your tissues.

As reviewed by Dr. Basil Wainwright, one of the world's leading practitioners and researchers in this field, "At the time when God first created man, man enjoyed an oxygen rich atmosphere of typically 38.2%. . . . Since that time, the oxygen content in the lower atmosphere has dropped from 23.9% prior to World War II, to presently 19.8% and lower in industrial/polluted environments. . . ." The ramifications of reduced environmental oxygen on human health "is severe indeed," Dr. Wainwright relayed to me from his post as AIDS science director for the country of Kenya. Included among the disastrous outcomes of this assault on God's oxygen rich planet, he said, "is a proliferation of anaerobic opportunistic infections" and increased cancer rates.

Several other factors contribute to oxygen depletion. Mineral deficiencies is one of them. Minerals help inhibit the formation of toxins in our soils, *and* the increase in toxins throws an extra burden on body oxygen levels. In addition, pollutants, overeating, stress, lack of exercise, infections, and improper breathing can cause increased need for oxygen. Researchers have also shown that fluoride in our drinking water slows down the process of oxidation of our foods. For all these reasons, supplementing your oxygen intake is being recommended by doctors, nutritionists, and other health professionals around the world.

In other words, even though oxygen saturation in the veins of modern man is 60-70%, some experts see a need for supplementing oxygen up to the 80-90% range.

Oxygenation, or infusing oxygen in one form or another into people for dramatic, even miraculous, health benefits, has virtually been practiced from the time God first breathed life into Adam. Today, oxygenation therapies include delivering oxygen into cells, tissues, and body organs through a variety of ways. The most common routes include nutritional supplementation in the form of food grade (35%) hydrogen peroxide, and magnesium peroxide, intravenous and rectal infusions of medical ozone, breathing higher percentages of environmental air oxygen generated by machines, and hyperbaric chamber delivery systems that force oxygen into your lungs and through your skin.

Antimicrobial Effects of Oxygenation

Most pathogenic microbes, including viruses, bacteria, and fungi, are anaerobic—they can't thrive in oxygen rich environments. Virtually every infectious disease epidemic owes its existence to oxygen deprivation more than to the germs widely blamed for the outbreaks.

Dr. Wainwright explains this phenomenon thusly: subatomic reactions occurring at the cellular level in response to oxidative reactions provide some "free radical" benefits. Included here are the "oxidization" of anaerobic microbes, foreign bodies, and cancerous growths and the deionization—that is, electrical discharging/inactivation—of positively charged infected cells within your body. Again, contrary to popular belief, not all "free radical" activity is bad. "Free radical" activity associated with oxidizing pathogenic microbes is clearly good.

Body Acidity, Free Radicals, Anti-Oxidants, and Oxygen

Some forms of oxygenation, including what Dr. Wainwright calls "Polyatomic Oxygen Therapy," has the ability to stimulate "cellular regenerative mechanisms" thereby accelerating your body's natural healing response.

All body systems, Dr. Wainwright reiterates, are electrochemically driven. Moreover, as I relayed in chapter 2, lowered blood pH can cause increased illness and growth of disease associated microbes. Recall that I included among acid risk factors virtually all drugs including antibiotics.

Technically, and more accurately, according to Dr. Wainwright, "an increase in blood level acidity, and increased 'electron transfer' activity (of 'free radicals'), is not *per se*, a bad thing, unless used excessively and consistently on a patient, which is a common feature of many pharmaceutical therapeutic preparations in medicine." Alternatively, the role of antioxidants, "actually increases the number of 'free radicals/electrons'" available to help protect the body. Likewise confusing, and opposite to what you might expect, Dr. Wainwright explains that "the consumption of vitamin C and citric acid will increase [y]our blood acidity levels. The result is that when a patient consumes anything which increases the acidity level in the bloodstream, one is actually allowing a more effective cellular 'electron transfer' ("free radicals"), to take place (similar to the reactions which occur in a car battery, whereupon charged electrons, which are stored in the lead plates of the battery, react with the sulfuric acid). Numerous scientific studies have established that an increase in acidity *combined with* an increase of 'Polyatomic Oxygen's hydroxyls and peroxyls in the bloodstream, will accelerate the eradication of diseased cells and dramatically reduce 'viral loads' in virally infected patients."

If this seems confusing to you, body acidity and "free radicals" being both *good and bad*, Dr. Wainwright offers clarification: Where doctors and physicians have genuine evidence of "free radical" problems in patients is in regard to "drifter molecules." These "drifter molecules" can be very dangerous to the human being, as these molecules can aggregate combinations of chlorine and fluorine atoms, generating serious health related complications if left unchecked. These "drifter molecules" can be a very unpleasant scourge in creating rheumatoid arthritic conditions.

"In fact," Dr. Wainwright concluded, under certain conditions, oxygenation therapies have been shown to "break down the bonding of the atoms in these 'drifter molecules.'"

Other scientific investigators showed that ozone can kill viral infected cells, disassociate, solubilize, and inactivate viruses as a result of ionization and/or oxidation, and inhibit viral "docking" to cells required for infection.

It should be understood that the ozone these scientists investigated and found helpful and healing bears no relationship to the "bad ozone" acknowledged to cause respiratory ailments. Their difference is clear. "Bad ozone" is commonly formed from industrial emissions, at low altitudes, as typically found in smog. In this case, low altitude O_3, produced by motor vehicles and industry, often becomes "trapped" when combined with sulfuric and nitric acid compounds in the air you breathe. This can increase your body acidity and cause the health problems previously described.

The Cancer Industry, Oxygenation, and the Blood "Banksters"

Likewise, it is the deprivation of "good ozone" and oxygen that has been linked for decades to cancer. Dr. Otto Warburg, the only scientist in history twice awarded the Nobel Peace Prize in Medicine, first proved cancer's direct link to low oxygen levels in the 1930s. "Cancer," he wrote, "above all other diseases, has countless secondary causes. Almost anything can cause cancer, but, even for cancer, there is only one prime cause. . . . the lack of cellular oxygen."

Dr. Warburg, like Dr. Wainwright, convinced of the safety, efficacy, and economy of oxygenation therapy, and troubled by the Rockefeller directed cancer monopoly, later wrote, "How long prevention will be avoided depends on how long the profits of agnosticism will succeed in inhibiting the application of scientific advancement and knowledge in the cancer field. In the mean time, millions of men and women must die of cancer unnecessarily."

Dr. Wainwright is a physicist who, prior to emigrating to Kenya, had been incarcerated in the United States for "practicing medicine without a license." He brilliantly treated and saved people using oxygenation therapies that were comparatively inexpensive and non-patentable. The cancer industrialists—the Rockefellers and their friends—decided to eliminate him as a competitive risk. These military–medical–industrialists would not look kindly upon the use of oxygen, not only to prevent infectious diseases and cure cancers, but clean up their contaminated blood supplies as well. Far more money can be made by spreading and "managing" diseases than by preventing and curing them.

This suppression of modern oxygenation technologies might make more sense following a review of the pertinent historic facts.

In the October 1, 1991 issue of the prestigious medical journal *Blood*, Dr. Bernard J. Poiesz, of the Department of Medicine at the State University of New York Health Science Center in Syracuse, while studying the AIDS virus, concluded "the effects of ozone include viral particle disruption, reverse transcriptase inactivation, and/or perturbation of the ability of the virus to bind to its receptor on target cells." He and his co-investigators, all affiliated with the Merck pharmaceutical company's manufacturing division, concluded, "Ozone treatment offers promise as a means to inactivate human retroviruses in human body fluids and blood product preparations." Despite this, to the time of this writing, the Food and Drug Administration (FDA) coupled with the Rockefeller directed blood banking industry, continue their negligence in allowing contaminated blood supplies to carry myriad viruses around the world to unwitting millions.

Parenthetically, and ironically, here is another bitter bit of medical history. It was this same Dr. Poiesz who vindicated Merck's experimental hepatitis B vaccine that came under widespread scientific suspicion as the international transmitter of the AIDS virus in the mid to late 1970s. Though the vaccine was given to gay men in New York City and Blacks in Central Africa, Poiesz's team neglected to study these populations for the apparent vaccine transmitted infection. As documented in *Emerging Viruses: AIDS & Ebola—Nature, Accident or Intentional?*, Dr. Poiesz's conflict of interest was shared by his intimate research colleague Dr. Robert Gallo. Dr. Gallo, readers of my earlier works might recall, is firmly linked to developing numerous AIDS-like viruses while directing one of America's leading biological weapons laboratories—Litton Bionetics. It was Litton that supplied Merck with the contaminated African chimpanzees used to make the suspected hepatitis B vaccine. Though Dr. Gallo had been investigated for scientific misconduct and/or fraud four times during the last part of the twentieth century, President Clinton pardoned him.

Thus, the "authorities" that likely spread AIDS and other blood borne pathogens around the world through contaminated vaccines and blood supplies, could have cleaned up the blood ages ago using oxygenation therapies, but they haven't. In essence, the Rockefeller family that monopolized American medicine in the early twentieth century, and funded the bogus Flexner investigation that vilified alternative therapies, also largely controls the American Red Cross, and continues to make vast fortunes from humanity's suffering with their spread of infectious agents throughout the world. Moreover, having monopolized world pharmaceutics in the 1930s in partnership with the infamous Nazi-linked IG Farben company, Rockefeller cohorts in the military–medical–pharmaceutical–industrial complex, including George W. Merck, president of the Merck pharmaceutical company, received the lion's share of the Nazi war chest at the close of WWII. Given Hilter's, Farben's, the Rockefeller's, and by association, Merck's links to "eugenics"— better known as "racial hygiene," or the "Human Genome Project," it is not likely a coincidence that the Rockefeller Foundation and Merck Fund are among the leading depopulation funding sources. Their current depopulation agenda, as published in the prestigious *Foreign Affairs* journal in March/April 1996, targets fifty percent of the American population for elimination. One of every two Americans must die according to a Rockefeller spin-off group called the Negative Population Growth, Inc. of New Jersey.

"Out of the question!" you might think. "Foolish conspiracy nonsense," you may wish to believe. But, if you have eyes to see the documentation, you may no longer be so naive. I've been saying for years now that their contaminated vaccines and blood supplies produce an insidious form of genocide. It was, after all, Laurance Rockefeller who put together the New York City blood council. That was the council of doctors who put together the New York City Blood Bank. These became the international blood "banksters." These are the people that allowed 10,000 hemophiliacs throughout the United States, and countless others around the world, to receive blood known to be contaminated with HIV between 1980 and 1986. The "banksters" did nothing significant to clean the blood. Easily done, they knew, using oxygenation technologies.

Same thing for Hepatitis C, which is most likely another man-made mutant of the original "Australian antigen" they now call Hepatitis B. Class action lawsuits are currently pending around the world concerning these blood delivered pathogens. The international blood "banksters" knew their blood shipments were contaminated with these agents, but they spread them anyway. The story is relayed in greater detail in *Emerging Viruses: AIDS & Ebola—Nature, Accident or Intentional?*

Bible Prophecy of Bio-Spiritual Warfare

The Bible (Ephesians 6:11-20) proclaims, "For our struggle is not against flesh and blood, but against the rulers, against the authorities, against the powers of this dark world and against the spiritual forces of evil in the heavenly realms. Therefore," you are counseled, "put on the full armor of God, so that when the day of evil comes you may be able to stand your ground, and after you have done everything . . . [S]tand firm then, with the belt of truth buckled around your waist, with the breastplate of righteousness in place, and with your feet fitted with readiness that comes from the gospel of peace." In chapter 7, I will share a true story about spiritual warfare surrounding a miracle that my daughter and I experienced in regard to "the belt of truth buckled around" our waists.

The Book of Revelation describes better than anything "end times" in which the kings and wealthiest men of all the nations were deceived by men who cast "spells" or practiced "sorcery." It warns against "evil . . . authorities," and "the powers of the dark world." The Rockefeller cohort clearly fit this description. Besides their great wealth and political power that reaches around the globe, the earliest word for "sorcery" is the Greek root word "pharmacopeia" or pharmacy. That may be correctly interpreted to mean the Rockefeller directed pharmaceutical industrialists have deceived international leaders. After all, the Rockefellers and their European counterparts, as discussed in *Healing Codes for the Biological Apocalypse*, largely control the International Monetary Fund (IMF). Their financial "spells" and pharmaceutical "sorcery" is not only associated in the Bible with the great plagues, it's linked to the onslaught of "beasts" as well.

In this "biospiritual warfare" allegory, the Bible prophesied beasts, along with plagues, famine, and war, are predicted to kill billions of people—ultimately about half of the world's population. Strikingly, this corresponds exactly to the published goal to reduce the U.S. population by half in the not-to-distant future.

Strong's Concordance root word for "beasts" is the Hebrew word (#2416) "chay" meaning "alive; having an appetite for raw flesh," like the flesh eating bacteria. And in the Greek Lexicon, the original word (#2342) for "beasts" is "therion" meaning "a little beast or little animal." That sounds like little bacteria and viruses as well.

As mentioned, the Rockefeller Foundation and the Merck Fund, that is, Merck, Sharp and Dohme—the world's leading vaccine manufacturer—are among the leading funding sources for world depopulation. Isn't it interesting that the Rockefellers largely control the pharmaceutical, blood, sterilization, and population control industries? Thus, the earth's greatest depopulation event is prophesied in Revelation to be associated with the little beasts and great plagues wielded like weapons by these "evil powers of the dark world." Clearly, the bacteria and viruses—infectious agents insidiously, precisely, and extensively spread in vaccines and contaminated blood—are bringing about Revelation's "end times" prophecy.

Finally, God's wrath in Revelation is predicted to be poured out largely because of these people and the masses who worship them. People who worship Babylon's idols get killed. My mother, for example, believed that M.D.s were Medical Deities. She unquestioningly followed her doctors' recommendations and got her flu vaccines. She died in 1992 of cancer in the wake of a disease commonly linked to flu vaccines—Guillain Barré. For this reason, I believe she was ultimately murdered. Given the Nazi links to the Rockefellers and Merck, I believe the people my mother escaped in Vienna in 1939, killed her in 1992.

Today, as modern medical science is idolized, and continues to dramatically alter the gene pools of plants, animals, bacteria, viruses, foods, and humans, the people who made vast fortunes during World War II continue to wreak havoc, play God, devastate populations, and make vast fortunes.

In *Healing Codes for the Biological Apocalypse*, Dr. Joseph Puleo and I explain, with stunning documentation, that "bio-spiritual warfare" is peaking at this extraordinary time in history. Bible prophecies are indeed being fulfilled. You better believe the Rockefellers and their friends are involved and control the world's blood banking, pharmaceutical, *and* oxygenation industries. They pull the political strings on the government agents and agencies that persecute people like Dr. Wainwright. They recognize that both blood and oxygen are critical requirements for conducting contemporary bio-spiritual warfare.

The Blood and the "Covenants of Promise"

Throughout the old testament, God's covenant with His chosen people depended on their following His commandments. When they failed to do so, that is, they sinned, God required the Israelites to restore their good faith by making food, animal, and blood sacrifices to the King of the Universe. As this strategy wasn't working well, that is, His people continued to sin, God's new plan in the "Covenants of Promise," (Ephesians 2:12) referred to the great hope in the shed *blood* of the Christ.

The word "covenant" is from the Hebrew word *bereat*, which means "to cut." This implies the shedding of *blood*. The reason blood is so important is because God knew of the life sustaining and spiritually uplifting power of blood. Thus, by His command and infinite grace, Yeshua's *blood* was shed, and made the vehicle for all atonement. Beginning with this sacrifice of the Messiah, whose blood would forever atone for the sins of all humanity, Christian gentiles were subsequently grafted into God's covenanted people.

"For the life of the flesh is in the blood," records Leviticus 17:11, "and I have given it to you on the altar, to make atonement for your souls. For it is the blood by reason of the life that makes atonement."

Later in this chapter you will learn more about "atonement." It implies more than "at-one-ment," or becoming one with God. In fact, by using the sound of His words in prayer you can join Him in the Holy Spirit. The spiritual dynamics and physics of what a "tone" really means will be detailed.

Thus, not only do the life sustaining properties of blood heal and keep you alive, but blood functions to bring about unity with God as well. The symbolic shedding of it by Yeshua, restored what Adam lost for Godkind. His sin imparted death, death implied mortality, mortality evidenced separation from God, but God's covenant and eternal grace now enables reunification with Him through the Holy Spirit. This is the most powerful and wonderful message delivered in this book.

It revolves around the sacred *blood*. The fact that humanity's blood is currently delivering horrific contaminants—infectious agents including "mad cow disease" prions, toxic fungi, and new immune-suppressive viral epidemics—is germane to the current waging of bio-spiritual warfare on humanity. Many of today's most lethal germs have been made and spread to alter human genetics and blood lines forever! Indeed, this too goes against God's laws and relates to Bible prophecy as you can read in Leviticus 19:19.

Throughout history, the secret societies that I write about in *Healing Codes for the Biological Apocalypse*, viewed blood as central to their nefarious achievements. Power mongers revered blood. Pagan and demonic rituals evolved around blood sacrifices for empowerment. Records memorialize the ceremonial drinking of blood from sacrificed animals and children in the quest for power. The search for the holy grail was conducted because it was believed to be filled with Yeshua's blood. This quest dominated the lives of knights, including the Knights Templar, their kings, including King James (from which the King James Version of the Bible originated), and other world leaders.

Likewise, today, blood holds the promise of temporal and extended salavation. Nazi scientists typed blood stolen from their captives, and then, depending on its judged "purity," blood was used as a means of granting extended life, or sentencing the persecuted to death. Relatedly, blood "worship" or "sacrifice" today is practiced in contemporary medicine, science, and even law. Practitioners in these fields look to reveal the secrets for extending life or, in the case of criminals identified through DNA blood analyses, to determine imprisonment or death. Blood bankers collect, freeze, and store blood in the event it is needed during life-threatening surgeries. Diets, science explains, should be predicated on *blood types.*

Red blood is made red due to its treasured passenger— *molecular oxygen.* It is, therefore, no accident that "blood work" and oxygen is central to all medical and healing procedures.

I've already discussed the fact that your white blood cells are central to your immune system, and function like a metaphor for self esteem and spiritual identity. The "God consciousness" within your "temple of God" precisely reflects the functioning immune system. White blood cells, you recall, are those that assess the difference between self and nonself, cancer cells versus normal cells, normal host proteins versus invading or infectious agents—bacteria, viruses, fungi, and more. So again, if you are estranged from God—lacking your spiritual identity—that is, you do not know who you are on the highest spiritual level, then your immune system cannot function optimally either. Your immune cells will simply be unable to recognize the difference between self and nonself.

Likewise, the red blood cells that carry oxygen to every cell in your body, virtually deliver God throughout your temple. As God breathed life into Adam, oxygen is central to spiritual healing and healthy human development.

Consider that the Hebrew name for God is "Yah-vah," which literally means "to breathe is to exist." To exist is to breathe! That is why many ancient names like Iss*iah*, Abr*ah*am, and my Hebrew name Ary*ah* include God's name. The greeting alo*ha* in Hawaiian, and *ah*sala*a*m in Arabic cultures, similarly declares God's presence. The "prana*[h]*" in Eastern religions, the energy of life, is carried by oxygen and inspired by deep abdominal breathing. It is well known that laughter facilitates healing. Why? Because the sound made during a belly laugh—"Ha h*ah*," or hearty yawn—"Ha*ah*h," replenishes the lungs, blood, and spirit. You know that laughter is generally contagious. People intimately long to be part of God and joyous celebrations. Indeed, calling out His name in hearty laughter is, in fact, bioelectrically transmissible. Others are compelled to yawn when they see you do it, because the spiritual affect of praising God with your laugh—"Ha, Ha, H*ah*," or yawn—"Haaa*ah*," travels magically through the ethers to uplift others who long for oxygen and God's Holy Spirit. Likewise, the sound that you make when you drop into a hot bath after a hard day gives praise to God—"Aaaaahhh!" Even a person's scream while under attack automatically calls God's name for Divine intercession—"A*ah*hhhhh!"

In summary, God's "covenant"—derived from the Hebrew word "bereat," which means to cut—implies the shedding of blood and oxygen. Just as "God formed a person . . . and breathed into his nostrils the breath of life, so that" he might be "a living being," God's grace is forever being poured into humanity, your body included, as oxygen literally inspires life. Likewise, God gave the world his Son, Yeshua, to effect his new covenant; to sacrifice the necessary blood to atone for humanity's sins. That was the ultimate gift of continuous grace and forgiveness. Like the oxygen God continuously provides, He is always willing to just forgive us if we simply and lovingly ask. Like any loving father, His hope is that we will just stop sinning, and return to His laws.

Remember, the root word for sin derives from the Greek archery term that means to be "off the mark." You're not in with the flow if you're sinning. You're not in line with the positive spiritual forces of God's great universe when you're not following His laws. And now, through faith in Him because of blessed Yeshua, your sin is always forgiven through His Divine sacrifice. So it's your blood and oxygen that carries with it the most vital spiritual essence. Given this significance alone, it is criminal that oxygenation technologies have been suppressed and kept from the manipulated masses.

Simple Forms of Oxygenation Therapy

What oxygenation strategies and therapies might you use? There are some simple things you can do to increase the amount of oxygen in your body such as incorporating aerobic exercise in your schedule. For instance, rebounding on mini-trampolines is an excellent way to bring more oxygen into your blood stream and stimulate your lymphatics. Another is making conscious decisions to take more full deep breaths throughout your day. You will find your posture improving as your chest expands when you inhale more completely. Many people reared in urban areas breathe too shallowly. This is understandable as it isn't desirable to inhale exhaust fumes and other pollutants in city air. So, if you are living in a city, and can afford to get out, do so NOW, or open an oxygen bar!

Another simple and inexpensive way to get more oxygen into your body is with 35% food grade hydrogen peroxide. This is available at most health food stores. However, this product is extremely strong and can burn skin. It needs to be used with caution. Don't confuse 35% food grade hydrogen peroxide with the 3% drug store variety that is used for wound cleaning. A few drops of the 35% food grade hydrogen peroxide diluted in purified drinking water, is excellent for increasing body oxygen content. People typically mix from four (4) to twenty-four (24) drops of this 35% solution in an eight (8) ounce glass of pure drinking water. Though this tastes *terrible*, many people feel it is a viable way to get more oxygen into your system, so long as the safety precautions are heeded.

The product *OxyAdvantage*™, as mentioned previously under fasting, is a pleasant-tasting low-priced alternative to marginally tolerating the above recipe. In fact, my family just loves its taste. This oxygenation product provides the equivalent of twenty-five (25) drops of 35% food grade hydrogen peroxide per one (1) ounce serving. *OxyAdvantage*™ has been meticulously manufactured with cold processed organic Aloe Vera as the carrier ingredient. The Aloe is saturated with oxygen that comes from magnesium peroxide, hydrogen peroxide, and choice herbal oxygenators. As an added value, the product provides a proprietary blend of immune boosting herbs and herbal extracts of Ginkgo Biloba, Hawthorne Berry, Ginseng, and St. John's Wort. These also increase oxygenation by helping to regulate heart rates. All benefits considered, this unique formula can help fight infections, degeneration, and inflammation while increasing your energy and mental alertness.

By the way, 35% food grade hydrogen peroxide is also good for preserving water. Since pure water in cities may be as valuable as gold in the future, it may be a good idea to have some stored. Only 2 drops of this form of hydrogen peroxide will preserve a gallon of water for months. I preserved a gallon of fresh water using this method, and after several months I was pleasantly surprised to find that it tasted as though it had just come out of a clean mountain stream.

This 35% food grade hydrogen peroxide can also be used to disinfect surfaces and items in the home and can even be used instead of toxic bleach as a whitener for your laundry.

Adding a quarter of a cup to a large bathtub of water and soaking in this oxygenating solution is also very rejuvenating and good to do if you happen to be sick or have any symptoms of a depressed immune system.

The "Koch Treatment"

William Frederick Koch is the man credited for having pioneered the use of oxygen in the treatment of such debilitating diseases as poliomyelitis, cancer, and even epilepsy. Dr. Koch held doctorates in biochemistry as well as in medicine. In the early 1930s, he discovered that homeopathic doses of oxidation catalysts, injected at cyclical intervals, supported oxidation mechanisms and facilitated natural immunity to disease. He also recommended a regimen of "fresh pure air, pure water, plenty of rest, and reasonable exercise" AND a diet of whole, natural foods—avoiding coffee, black tea, chocolate, refined sugars, alcohol, and tobacco. He published this in 1939 in his book entitled, *The Chemistry of Natural Immunity*. Subsequently, thanks to the suppressive monopolistic practices of the Rockefeller directed FDA persecutors, "the Koch treatment," what these injections of oxidation catalysts became known as, became illegal in the United States.

A friend of mine told me her experience using Koch treatments that were given to her in Los Angeles in the 1950s by a doctor who had to send to Switzerland for the product. She had asthma, and had just experienced a severe attack brought on by an unusually stressful experience. The doctor gave her an injection of these Koch catalysts, and within a few hours she experienced a sense of euphoria and well-being. She found herself breathing deeply and having several loose bowel movements a day as though her body were discharging toxins. As a result of this treatment, her asthma completely disappeared and has never returned.

Hyperbaric Oxygenation

Today there are hyperbaric oxygenation chambers available, typically associated with medical clinics, throughout the world. You can also purchase portable units for less than $5,000 (U.S.). If you think that's a lot of money, let me relay one woman's story.

One afternoon, following a presentation I made during a health conference in which I mentioned oxygenation therapies, a middle-aged woman approached me with her success story. She allegedly needed knee surgery. She couldn't walk comfortably anymore and limped severely. She went to a physician, who referred her to a surgeon. The surgeon gave her a treatment plan estimated to cost between $25–30,000 (U.S.). She asked, "Isn't there anything else I can do?" He told her, "Well, I don't know. You can check around." So she sought and found another physician who told her he could treat the same condition successfully using oxygenation. He told her, "I think you're going to get major benefits, but I can't guarantee it."

"How much is it going to cost?" she asked.

"Five treatments will cost $5,000," he returned.

She bought his services and I saw her results. She was walking virtually back to normal.

So you can purchase your own unit, keep it in your home, and treat yourself, your family, and all of your friends for the cost of one patient's medical expense.

Air Oxygenation Machines

Also available on the market are some very good oxygenation aeration units. Alpine Air, for example, sells an excellent unit for about $650 (U.S.). That's their top of the line machine.

A less expensive unit, but also highly effective is called the Aranizer. It is the highest quality, lowest cost, unit that I have found. I have two small units at home operating all the time in our bedroom and my office. They cost about $250 (U.S.) dollars each. The larger Aranizer model, for $450 (U.S.), disinfects, ionizes, and treats up to 5,000 cubic feet of air.

These units are ideal for oxygenating homes and small workplaces. They effectively oxygenate between 1,000 and 5,000 cubic feet fairly rapidly. You can actually feel the difference within minutes of turning them on. They are ideal for bedroom usage while sleeping because that's a great time for healing. When you put one of these units in your bedroom, you will feel like you're sleeping next to a babbling brook which is throwing off little water particles that have been aerated. That's what it tastes like, smells like, and feels like when you use a good machine. If you buy a machine that doesn't do this for you, return it.

Most of these devices produce negative air ions. In the environment, negative air ions get rid of anaerobic bacteria, molds, and fungi. Those germs, along with other air pollutants including smoke and dust particles, are typically positively charged. Generated negative air ions, through electromagnetic attraction, connect with the positive pollutant ions and neutralize their charge. As a result, they largely fall to the floor where you can vacuum or sweep them up along with other house dust. With this benefit, besides getting additional oxygen into your lungs throughout the day and night, these machines can be absolutely lifesaving for asthmatics, and extremely helpful for people who suffer with allergies.

Chlorophyll for Blood Loss Victims

Last, but not least, particularly for accident victims who lose a lot of blood, the need for oxygen is critical. Drinking chlorphyll may be life-saving. Chlorophyll can be used as a pint for pint blood replacement. Likewise, for anemics, this recommendation is most important. Get a bottle of chlorophyll from your health food store. Drinking it as a substutute for blood transfusion has saved many people from this unwanted and/or unwarranted medical intervention which, thanks to blood "bankster" negligence and corruption, remains very risky.

Chapter 6.
Bioacoustics and Electromedicine: God's Healing Technologies

"There are undoubtedly all kinds of sounds in the world, and none is altogether meaningless; . . . These are the things we are talking about when we avoid the manner of speaking that human wisdom would dictate and instead use a manner of speaking taught by the Spirit."

1 Corinthians 14:10 and 2:13,
The Holy Bible

A nother royally suppressed area is electromedicine. This includes the brilliant work of Royal Raymond Rife and his genius mentor, Nikola Tesla.

Star Trek fans rejoiced when "Bones" waved a little electrical device over Captain Kirk's ailing body and, seconds later, his wounds were healed. That's close to where we would be in healing practice if it wasn't for the Rockefeller directed medical-monopolists who have been suppressing the entire field of electromedicine since the early 1900s.

Now this aggravates me. It would also disturb you if you were to read *The Science of Coercion* (Oxford University Press, 1994) by Christopher Simpson, which I reference in *Emerging Viruses: AIDS & Ebola—Nature, Accident or Intentional?* Simpson studied psychological warfare methods used on health scientists and health professionals from 1945 to virtually the present. He concluded that if you were a scientist or healthcare professional who did not follow the Rockefeller directed medical/pharmaceutical agenda, then you were traditionally demoted, defunded, and ostracized. Those who kept bucking the system were persecuted and often jailed like Dr. Brezynski in Texas, Dr. Beljenski in France, Dr. Wainwright now in Kenya, and countless others that have been arrested for providing successful, low cost, low risk therapies. That, Simpson concludes, is how control has been maintained all these years.

So numerous healthcare professionals have needed to go "underground" to use alternative technologies, nutritional supplements, oxygenation, and/or electromagnetic therapies. Otherwise, they risk being arrested or losing their medical licenses.

What branch of the "medical mafia" enforces this madness in the name of "public health and safety?" Who makes the arrests and persecutes healthcare's brightest leading humanitarians? The FDA, that's who.

Now think about whether this makes sense. The FDA puts all the costly and risky AIDS and cancer drugs on their "fast track" for testing and approval. They approve brand new vaccines, poorly tested at best, even though most of them deliver a whole assortment of autoimmune disease inducing agents. They neglect or downplay vaccine risks such as chronic fatigue and fibromyalgia, lupus, MS, ALS, crippling rheumatoid arthritis, type-1 diabetes, autism, asthma, hayfever and allergies, AIDS, Gulf War Syndrome, meningitis, Alzheimer's, autism, and sudden infant death syndrome (SIDS). Their officials pay little attention to the science linking contaminated vaccines, or blood supplies, that these people approve as "safe," to these raging iatrogenic epidemics. In essence, the FDA, who literally regulates 25% of the United States economy today, puts toxic waste on a silver platter for drug company profit and legislative demand! Yet, they work to regulate and remove natural healing alternatives—take away your over-the-counter vitamins and herbs, and outlaw health food store botanicals and supplements.

Excuse me! Is there something wrong with this picture?

Behind the scenes in this effort to limit or eliminate your access to vitamins, minerals, herbs, and other natural low-risk supplements is the German-based legislation now pending at the Rockefeller directed World Health Organization (WHO) called Codex Alimentarius. This legislation, if passed, will make it far more costly and difficult, if not impossible, for you to purchase preventative nutritional supplements without a prescription from a licensed medical doctor.

Electromagnetics and Divine Healing Technologies

A more uplifting direction was exemplified by blessed Yeshua when, after a forty-day fast, he implemented God's magnificent healing ministry. How does the Father and His Son continue to perform miracles for those who place their faith and trust in them? How was Yeshua able to touch people and have them miraculously heal? How does God heal? When you go to sleep at night feeling sick and tired, why do you wake up in the morning feeling so refreshed?

The answers to all of these questions lies in the multidisciplinary study of physics, genetics, biochemistry, mathematics, language, electromagnetism, spirituality, and scripture. Through electromagnetics—God's technology underlying spirituality and Divine healing—all of the above miracles are possible and even largely explained.

Electromagnetism is defined in *Webster's Dictionary* as "a fundamental physical force that is responsible for interactions between charged particles which occur because of their charge and for the emission and absorption of photons [light energy] . . ." Thus, strictly adhering to its definition, since every physical object is composed of atoms and subatomic particles that interact because of electromagnetic phenomena, one might say that electromagnetism is fundamentally responsible for all life, and everything in the physical universe. It is also akin to the ether—the spiritual force or energy—that gives rise to all matter.

Take oxygen for example. As mentioned previously, every aspect of life depends on this element. Energizing every function in your body through the Krebs (tricarboxylic acid) cycle, oxygen plays a critical role in freeing up ATPs—your body's main electromagnetic energy rich molecule. This is the end toward which carbohydrate, fat, and protein metabolism all point, that is, the production of more electromagnetic energy.

Another relationship between oxygen and electromagnetic energy exists in the formation of ozone. Oxygen (0_2) normally absorbs ultraviolet light radiation. This initiates a chemical reaction which creates ozone.

Furthermore, oxygen's root words according to *Webster's Dictionary* are *oxy*—relating to "sharp, acid," and *gen*—pertaining to "information . . . producer; . . . born and become," forms the majority of water molecules. Recent research shows that water molecules have an electromagnetic energy storing capability. This frequency memory is thought to be associated with water's molecular structure composed of two oxygen atoms combined with one atom of hydrogen.

The shape of a water molecule simulates the structure of a tetrahedron—the most stable structure in the physical universe. These four sided equilateral triangular pyramids of water hold Divine symmetry. Using sacred geometry, they are able to receive, store, and transmit electromagnetic energy and healing frequencies.

This electromagnetic memory absorption and transmission capacity of oxygen and water largely explains how homeopathic solutions work. In essence, homeopathic medicines only contain water, a little alcohol for sterility and stability, and nothing else except the electromagnetic frequency of the disease "nosode" passed on through serial dilutions to the final product.

Likewise, medicinal herbs transmit their own specific electromagnetic frequencies for healing, as do essential oils. Both are prescribed throughout the Bible.

In addition to storing and transmitting electromagnetic frequencies, water (as well as cells and tissues) can be structurally altered by electromagnetic energy frequencies of sound, light, and even prayer, according to leading water researchers. Thus, the association between sound, light, prayer, and healing, on all levels, begins with oxygen and water.

Similarly, that is how spiritual "hands-on" healers promote recovery, and how Yeshua was able to produce miraculous healings. They transmit God's healing energy into people through spirit, oxygen, and water molecules coursing throughout their bodies.

It is well known that radio and television signals are carried by specific electromagnetic frequencies. This involves transmitting, channeling, and receiving electromagnetic energy. In the case of healing, it is God's Holy Spirit that is being transmitted. The Holy Spirit is the source, if not the channel, for Divine healing. As you will learn in the next section, water molecules surrounding cellular DNA absorb, recall, and transmit this healing Spirit to their surroundings.

In theory, and much successful practice of homeopathy and electromedicine, every disease state and pathogen has its associated harmonic and disharmonic frequencies. Generally speaking, harmonic frequencies maintain health, promote growth and healing, while discordant frequencies produce stress, illness, and death.

Clustered Water

Incredibly, harmonic frequencies of electromagnetic radiation can transform water molecules into hexagonal rings called *clustered water.* Flash frozen, these six-sided molecular structures resemble beautiful crystalline snow flakes as seen in figure 6.1.

Fig. 6.1. 20,000 Magnification of Flash Frozen Water

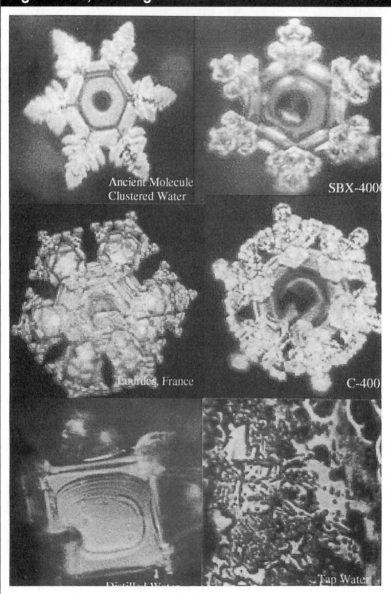

20,000 magnification photographs of different cryogenically prepared (i.e., flash frozen) water clusters. Upper left is ancient polar sample taken from two miles beneath the polar ice cap indicative of God's most pristine water. Middle left photo shows clustered water sample taken from the healing well at Lourdes France. Upper and middle right are similar clustered water molecules developed by Dr. Lee Lorenzen. Lower left and right are similarly prepared samples of distilled and tap water, respectively. Courtesy of CellCore International (949-261-7788).

Dr. Lee Lorenzen, one of the world's leading experts in clustered water technology, and his co-investigators, discovered that these *crystal*-shaped hexagonal clustered water molecules form the supportive *matrix* of healthy DNA. These clustered water molecules activate the genetic sequence's ability to receive and transmit electromagnetic signals—what Nobel Peace Prize in Medicine winners have termed "photon-phonon emissions for intercellular communications."

In fact, during the 1990s, three Nobel prize winners in medicine advanced research that revealed the primary function of DNA lies not in protein synthesis, as was widely believed, but in electromagnetic energy reception and transmission. Less than three percent of DNA's function is in protein formulation; more than ninety percent functions in the realm of bioelectric signaling.

During aging and intoxication, these DNA supportive water clusters are depleted. This compromises the electrical potential, integrity, reception, and signaling capacity of your DNA. This, Dr. Lorenzen and others believe, is the primary process underlying aging.

According to biochemist and author Steve Chemiske, these hexagonal shaped water rings supporting the DNA double helix, "vibrate at specific resonant frequencies and these frequencies can help restore homeostasis to cell structures in the body through signal transduction . . . the process by which one form of energy is converted to another.

"When clustered water is consumed, high frequency information is transmitted to proteins . . . [and] this wave of information is carried throughout the body like a 'wake-up call' to restore normal function."

Dr. Franco Bistolfi, a bioelectronics expert, theorized that intercellular communications, instantaneously affecting cells throughout the body, occurs "by means of piezoelectric interac-

Fig. 6.2. Cover of *TIME*'s Future of Medicine Issue

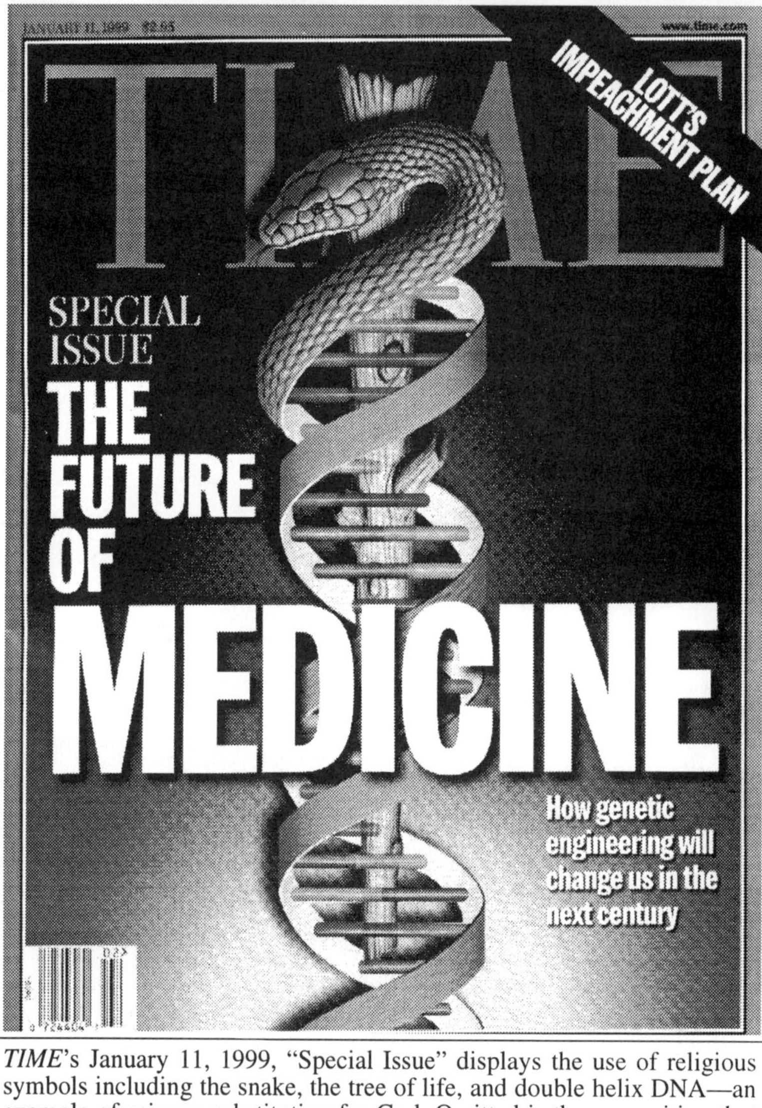

TIME's January 11, 1999, "Special Issue" displays the use of religious symbols including the snake, the tree of life, and double helix DNA—an example of science substituting for God. Omitted is the recognition that the primary function of DNA is spiritual. Genes are surrounded by clustered water molecules that facilitate "photon–phonon transmissions" of electromagnetic energies to up-regulate the functions of cells and tissues. Thus, vibrations are transmitted through DNA for "good" or "evil."

tions and photon/phonon transduction of electromagnetic signals of both endogenous and exogenous origin."

In other words, tiny imperceptible electromagnetic signals, both man-made and natural, harmonic or disharmonic, profoundly influence the oxygen and water molecules supporting DNA, health status, or alternatively, the pathogenic processes involved in virtually every disease.

It's extraordinary that Revelation predicted that the Messianic Age, and great "healing of the nations," would be accompanied by "crystal clear water" flowing through the "rivers and streams" in light of evolving research in DNA and clustered water. These "rivers and streams," Revelation revealed, are "the people." It is remarkable that the structure upholding the "tree of life"—DNA—as seen in figure 6.2, is not a snake, but, in reality, pure water clusters. In its healthy state, the crystal cluster supported double helix acts as an electromagnetic energy receiver and transmitter. Scientists now believe this is the primary function of DNA.

Moreover, the structure of more than 4,000 enzymes that regulate virtually every body function largely depends on these same hexagonal-shaped water clusters.

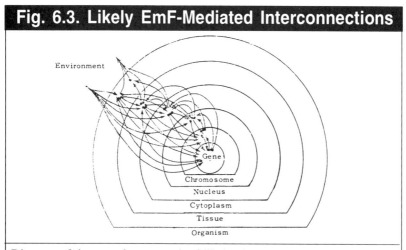

Fig. 6.3. Likely EmF-Mediated Interconnections

Diagram of the complex network of likely electromagnetic field and frequency interactions in living organisms. Initially hypothesized by A. S. Presman in *Electromagnetic Fields and Life*, (New York: Plenum Press, 1970, p. 243), recent scientific discoveries are confirming Presman's thesis.

Electromagnetic Frequencies and Gene Functions

In the definitive textbook on *Electromagnetic Fields and Life* (Plenum Press, 1970), by Russia's top biophysicist, Dr. A.S. Pressman, the works of numerous scientists investigating electromagnetic frequencies and genetic functions are discussed. Pressman provided the diagram seen in figure 6.3 depicting the "complex network of possible interactions in organisms" between DNA and up-regulation of the entire organism by way of electromagnetic transmissions. As seen in the figure, genetic electromagnetic signals communicate regulatory messages from the gene and chromosome through the nucleus, cell cytoplasm, body tissues, and ultimately to the entire organism and its environment. As shown, this signaling can also occur in reverse, that is, from the environment, or the Holy Spirit, to the gene core of every cell in your body.

As Pressman described it:

> If the described effects are considered from the standpoint of the concept of diverse EmF [electromagnetic field] interactions within the organisms and its interactions with environmental EmFs, then we can sketch a picture which is very convincing in its simplicity and consistency. In fact, we can picture the organism provided with diverse interconnections of such kind (in addition, of course, to the known diverse neurohumoral [nerve and hormonal] connections), differentiated as regards their specific "working" frequencies, intensity ranges, and method of coding. Such interconnections may underlie not only the interactions between cells, but also specific interactions between macromolecules: enzyme and substrate, antigen and antibody, DNA and RNA. Similar interconnections may be responsible for the control of protein synthesis. In a recently proposed hypothesis regarding such control, . . . DNA molecules are regarded as generators of radio-frequency signals, RNA molecules as amplifiers, and enzymes and amino acids as effectors of signals coded in various regions of the spectrum; the cell wall is believed to act as a noise filter.

Thus, reflecting on the Nobel Prize winning research in the 1990s, twenty years after Pressman wrote the above hypothesis, it's certain his theory is being supported by evolving science in the fields of genetics, biochemistry, and biophysics.

Creation Through Sound Vibration

Of all the articles on the powerful influence vibrational frequencies have on physical matter, a German investigator, Peter Pettersson, provided one of the best. In "Cymatics: The Science of the Future?", he effectively summarized the creative connection between sound, vibrations, and physical reality as he reviewed the work of the field's top researchers. Pettersson laid the foundation for scientifically comprehending creationism. This was also discussed in *Healing Codes for the Biological Apocalypse*.

Pettersson began with Ernst Chladni, the first observer of the "Chladni figures"—the shapes and forms produced as a result of sound vibrations striking the surface of matter. Chladni was, not surprisingly, a musician and physicist. Born in 1756, he laid the foundations for the discipline within physics called acoustics— the science of sound.

In 1787, Chladni published *Entdeckungen über die Theorie des Klanges* or *Discoveries Concerning the Theory of Music*. "In this and other pioneering works he explained ways to make sound waves generate visible structures. With the help of a violin bow which he drew perpendicularly across the edge of flat plates covered with sand," Pettersson wrote, Chladi "produced those patterns and shapes which today go by the term Chladni figures." This was significant because it demonstrated that sound actually affected physical matter. It held the power to create geometric forms in substances.

Later, in 1815, Nathaniel Bowditch—an American mathematician who followed up on Chladni's work—studied "the patterns created by the intersection of two sine curves whose axes are perpendicular to each other, sometimes called "Bowditch curves," but more often "Lissajous figures," . . . after the French mathematician Jules-Antoine Lissajous who, independently of Bowditch, investigated them in 1857-58. Both concluded that the condition for these designs to arise was that the frequencies, or oscillations per second, of both curves stood in simple whole-number ratios to each other, such as 1:1, 1:2, 1:3, and so on. In fact, one can produce Lissajous figures even if the frequencies are not in perfect, but close, whole-number rations to each other. If the difference is insignificant, *the phenomenon that arises is that the designs keep changing* their appearance." This, knowledge, applied to electromedicine, as you will soon learn, provides tremendous potential for healing virtually every illness.

Such figures, transformed by fluctuating frequencies, shift and change. What created the variations in the shapes of these designs was "the phase differential, or the angle between the two curves. In other words, the way in which their rhythms or periods," their harmonics, coincided or not determined the shaping and movement of physical structures. Likewise, pertaining to healing once again, harmonious or discordant frequencies have been shown to produce striking differences in human tissues.

In 1967, Hans Jenny, a Swiss physician and researcher, published in his native language *The Structure and Dynamics of Waves and Vibrations*. Jenny, like Chladni two-hundred years earlier, showed what happened when one took various materials like water, sand, iron filings, spores, and viscous substances, and placed them on membranes and vibrating metal plates. Shapes and patterns in motion appeared that varied from "perfectly ordered and stationary" to those that were chaotic.

Pettersson acknowledged Jenny for originating the field of "cymatics" that allowed people to observe the physical results of voice, tones, and song. Jenny applied the name "cymatics," from the Greek term "kyma," meaning "wave," to this area of re-

Fig. 6.4. Cymatics of Hebrew Sounds Forming Their Respective Letter Shapes

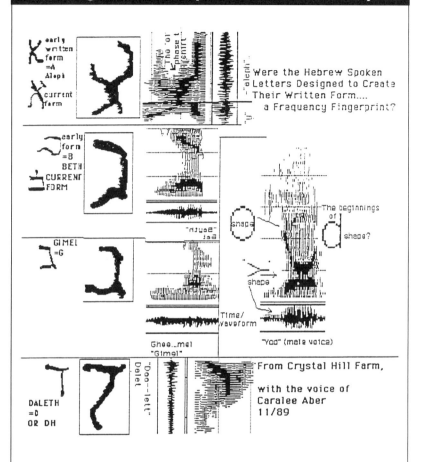

A Frequency Picture Alphabet..

... Speaking of the Shape of Sound.

11/89

In observing these spectral pictures of our alphabet...

Diagram shows "frequency fingerprints" of the first four Hebrew alphabet letters spoken into frequency registration graphing equipment. "Frequency Picture Alphabet" graphs of letters Aleph, Beth, Gimel, and Daleth are shown formed from their spoken tones. Source: S. Tenen and D. Winter in "A Personal Journey into the Truth," A self-published workbook, 1998, by J. Puleo.

search. Thus, cymatics could be defined as: "The study of how vibrations generate and influence patterns, shapes, and moving processes."

In addition, using his tonoscope, Jenny "noticed that *when the vowels of the ancient languages of Hebrew and Sanskrit were pronounced, the sand took the shape of the written symbols for these vowels.*" Modern languages, including English, failed to generate these patterns.

American researchers confirmed Jenny's findings. Stan Tenen and Dan Winter reproduced the effects using the Hebrew alphabet. They concluded that the "sacred languages" were indeed sacred in this way. Figure 6.4 shows a sample of their research. *This knowledge lays the foundation for understanding creationism in the strict sense from God's spoken word* as detailed in the Book of Genesis.

In summary, before I relay more on language, creationism, and healing, Jenny provided examples of cymatic elements found throughout nature—"vibrations, oscillations, pulses, wave motions, pendulum motions, rhythmic courses of events, serial sequences, and their effects and actions." These, he concluded, affected everything including biological evolution. *The evidence convincingly demonstrated that all natural phenomena were ultimately dependent on, if not entirely determined by, the frequencies of vibration.* According to Pettersson, Jenny "speculated that every cell had its own frequency, and that a number of cells with the same frequency created a new frequency which was in harmony with the original, which in its turn possibly formed an organ that also created a new frequency in harmony with the two preceding ones." Regarding healing, Jenny argued that recovery from disease states could be aided or hindered by tones. Just as Presman theorized, and modern science supports, Jenny believed that different frequencies influenced genes, cells, and various structures in the body.

Fig. 6.5. Derivation of English Letter Number Values

Letter & Number	Pythagorean Skein Equivalent	Key Word Number Derivations
A 1	1	T 20–2 + 0 = 2
B 2	2	R 18–1 + 8 = 9
C 3	3	U 21–2 + 1 = 3
D 4	4	S 19–1 + 9 = 1
E 5	5	T 20–2 + 0 = 2
F 6	6	98=8 17=8
G 7	7	
H 8	8	
I 9	9	F 6–6 + 0 = 6
J 10	1 + 0 = 1	A 1–1 + 0 = 1
K 11	1 + 1 = 2	I 9–9 + 0 = 9
L 12	1 + 2 = 3	T 20–2 + 0 = 2
M 13	1 + 3 = 4	H 8–8 + 0 = 8
N 14	1 + 4 = 5	44=8 26=8
O 15	1 + 5 = 6	
P 16	1 + 6 = 7	G 7–7 + 0 = 7
Q 17	1 + 7 = 8	O 15–1 + 5 = 6
R 18	1 + 8 = 9	D 4–4 + 0 = 4
S 19	1 + 9 = 10	26=8 17=8
T 20	2 + 0 = 2	
U 21	2 + 1 = 3	**The number 8**
V 22	2 + 2 = 4	**represents infinity.**
W 23	2 + 3 = 5	**9 represents**
X 24	2 + 4 = 6	**completion**
Y 25	2 + 5 = 7	
Z 26	2 + 6 = 8	

Table shows the English alphabet and its equivalent numbers. Two or more digit numbers are reduced to single digit numbers to employ the Pythagorean skein and determine the mathematical "truth." Notice that numbers one through nine repeat; and the number 8, the universal sign for "infinity," is also the total for "Trust," "Faith" and "God." The number nine (9) represents completion.

Cathie E. Guzetta, a poet, summarized this science when she wrote, "The forms of snowflakes and faces of flowers may take on their shape because they are responding to some sound in nature. Likewise, it is possible that crystals, plants, and human beings may be, in some way, music that has taken on visible form."

Trust, Faith, God, and Alphanumerics

In *Healing Codes for the Biological Apocalypse*, my colleague, Dr. Joseph Puleo, relayed how mathematics, the most precise language, is "God's language" because it always speaks the truth. Through Divine guidance he learned, as Hans Jenny had observed, that the Hebrew language, as well as English backwards, held a spiritual relationship through their alphanumeric translation.

In brief, Dr. Puleo took the English alphabet, from A to Z, as seen in figure 6.5, and numbered each letter. For example, A=1, B=2, C=3, and so on.

After this, he was instructed to take the words "TRUST," "FAITH," and "GOD," and perform a mathematical translation on them.

For "TRUST," T=20 + R=18 + U=21, + S=19, and T=20 totals 98. Then he used the ancient Pythagorean mathematics method of reducing each number to a single digit. So 9+8=17; then finally, 1+7=8.

You get the same result—"8"—when you decipher the numerical equivalent of each letter first, then add their total according to the Pythagorean skein. The same thing occurs with the words "FAITH" and "GOD."

For "FAITH," F=6, A=1, I=9, T=20, and H=8 totals 44. And 4+4=8.

For "GOD," G=7, O=15, and D=4 totals 26. And again 2+6=8.

Eight (8), he realized is the sign of infinity, that is, "God's number." Interestingly enough, it is also the number for oxygen in the periodic elemental table.

Any way you add them according to Pythagorean mathematics the words "TRUST," "FAITH" and "GOD" always add up to 8!

These, along with many other revelations, convinced Dr. Puleo that language was integrated with mathematics, and encoded with electromagnetic frequencies of sound that, as Jenny concluded relayed spiritual messages between people, and between people and God as well.

"Ultimately," Dr. Puleo concluded, "You can't take mathematics, or even science, out of God, or God out of science, because that leaves you with only half the picture."

The Alphanumerics, Holy Spirit, and Power of Language

Knowing there was something sacred about the number eight (8), and knowing, according to the Bible, God always multiplies and never adds numbers, Dr. Puleo deciphered all multiples of eights reduced to their Pythagorean single digit integer beginning with $1 \times 8 = 8$; $2 \times 8 = 16$ where $1 + 6 = 7$; $3 \times 8 = 24$ where $2 + 4 = 6$; and so on as seen in figure 6.6. He then realized the multiples of 8 produced a numerical countdown pattern—8, 7, 6, 5, 4, 3, 2, 1, 9, 8, 7, 6, 5, 4, 3, 2, 1, 9, 8, 7, 6, 5, 4, 3, 2, 1 which corresponded to the alphanumerics of the English language *backwards*! More incredibly, as shown in the figure, if you sum the alphanumeric equivalents of the English alphabet forwards added to backwards, the Pythagorean integer that always results is nine (9)—the number associated with "completion" and "OXYGEN."

Now let's say you were the German descended Anglo-Saxon, and later Norman, ruling elite who developed this spiritually reversed or mathematically compromised English language between 500 to 1,000 years after Christ's death. Let's also theorize

Fig. 6.6. Column Showing Multiples of Eights (8)

Multiple of Eights	Reverse Alphabet	Alphabet w/ Numbers	Sum of Two Alphabet #s
1 X 8 = 0 8 —— 8	Z	A 1	9
2 X 8 = 1 6 —— 7	Y	B 2	9
3 X 8 = 2 4 —— 6	X	C 3	9
4 X 8 = 3 2 —— 5	W	D 4	9
5 X 8 = 4 0 —— 4	V	E 5	9
6 X 8 = 4 8 —— 3	U	F 6	9
7 X 8 = 5 6 —— 2	T	G 7	9
8 X 8 = 6 4 —— 1	S	H 8	9
9 X 8 = 7 2 —— 9	R	I 9	9
1 0 X 8 = 8 0 —— 8	Q	J 1	9
1 1 X 8 = 8 8 —— 7	P	K 2	9
1 2 X 8 = 9 6 —— 6	O	L 3	9
1 3 X 8 = 1 0 4 —— 5	N	M 4	9
1 4 X 8 = 1 1 2 —— 4	M	N 5	9
1 5 X 8 = 1 2 0 —— 3	L	O 6	9
1 6 X 8 = 1 2 8 —— 2	K	P 7	9
1 7 X 8 = 1 3 6 —— 1	J	Q 8	9
1 8 X 8 = 1 4 4 —— 9	I	R 9	9
1 9 X 8 = 1 5 2 —— 8	H	S 1	9
2 0 X 8 = 1 6 0 —— 7	G	T 2	9
2 1 X 8 = 1 6 8 —— 6	F	U 3	9
2 2 X 8 = 1 7 6 —— 5	E	V 4	9
2 3 X 8 = 1 8 4 —— 4	D	W 5	9
2 4 X 8 = 1 9 2 —— 3	C	X 6	9
2 5 X 8 = 2 0 0 —— 2	B	Y 7	9
2 6 X 8 = 2 0 8 —— 1	A	Z 8	9

Column of multiples of eights (8) deciphered according to the Pythagorean skein in which all integers are reduced to single digits using addition of each digit in the whole number. Example: 208=2+0+8=10; then 10=1+0=1. This number is associated with the letter A. When A=1 is added to the reverse alphabet letter Z=8, the sum is 9. The number nine (9) implies completion and results everytime the numerical equivalents to letters are similarly added.

your secret society and royalty were very knowledgeable about spirituality, and like the Levi priests of old, understood the Pythagorean skein of mathematics and its relevance to spiritual and electromagnetic forces. Let's also assume you created this language, and hid the truth about its mathematical origins, in an effort manipulate the masses. That you had the awareness of the power of God, and that you knew the love of God was inherent in the original languages. But you had the evil desire to share an alternate fraudulent language with the public so that they would remain ignorant of, and distanced from, spiritual Divinity.

Given the above likelihood, by creating a new language through a mathematical code, you would never want to lose the original code to recover the original spiritually empowered language. So likely, at best, you would bury the code in an obvious place so that it would never be lost, but only accessed by knowledgeable associates who shared your secret desires.

This is what we relay in *Healing Codes for the Biological Apocalypse*. Naturally it relates to the story in the Bible that discusses the confusion of languages. This "Tower of Babel" story begins in Genesis 11:1. It reads, "Now the whole world had one language and a common speech." Using the common speech, language, and sounds, Godly empowered people who followed *His Word*, were blessed and nurtured. Soon, however, they became self-centered Godless pagans. They successfully built a "tower" that reached into the heavens. "But the Lord came down to see the city and the tower that the men were building. The Lord said, 'If as one people speaking the same language they have begun to do this, then nothing they plan to do will be impossible for them.'" (See Genesis 11:5-6.) So God decided to act decisively, creating the model that would later be used by the Anglo-Saxon/English ruling elite in their attempt to control the world through colonialism and language. In Genesis 11:7, God moved to destroy the earliest Babylonian rulers' plan. "Come," the Father said, "let us go down and confuse their language so they will not understand each other." So, "the Lord scattered them from there over all the earth, and they stopped building the city."

Clearly there is strength in unity, and God, very apparently, did not want Godless, evil, egomaniacal, pagans to become powerful earthly rulers. So by His *word* he scattered them around the earth by manipulating their speech, which, much like His powerful word, is sound conveying electromagnetic frequencies that powerfully influence physical matter.

Thus, through the introduction of foreign tongues, people could no longer understand one another. You had the loss of the edified congregation. Then, fear and hate took over. Later, with the introduction of still more languages, instead of speaking sacred and spiritually uplifting "tongues" (such as Hebrew and Sanscrit) wherein the tones of the spoken words actually relayed a Spiritual essence; that is, harmonic sounds that delivered health and vitality through the Holy Spirit, other mathematically derived languages were created that caused disharmony and discord. Thus, increasingly, humans beings were distanced from each other, as was humanity from God.

As it was then, so it is today, God breaks contact and withdraws His protection, and nurturing, from those who do not speak His language. His Holy language is based on mathematics, truth, justice, order, and humility attained through Godly praise and prayer while following His commandments and word.

Of course, you may recall, in the beginning there was only God and His word. Nothing else existed according to Genesis 1:1. Many scientists and Bible scholars believe that God and His word are inseparable. For all practical purposes, they are the same. One such theorist is Dr. Sir Peter Guy Manners, among the world's leading experts in cymatics. Dr. Manners argues that the electromagnetic frequencies of sound and words project powerful messages and forces through creative ether that clearly alter matter's form and function.

God spoke the universe into existence in *six* days. Jericho's great wall was shattered by seven Levi priests who encircled the city, likewise, for *six* days. Each day they shook the wall with the sounds played through their rams horns. So electromagnetic frequencies of sound clearly can be used for creation, destruction, and producing miracles.

Additionally, at this unique time in history, our Father wishes you to understand this power in His and your spoken words. He wants you to know that since words can be used to create, destroy, and produce miracles, they can, and are, used for good and evil by good and bad men alike. As Yeshua counseled us in Matthew 12:34-36:

> "For out of the overflow of the heart the mouth speaks. The good man brings good things out of the good stored up in him, and the evil man brings evil things out of the evil stored up in him. But I tell you that men will have to give account on the day of judgment for every careless word they have spoken. For by your words you will be acquitted, and by your words you will be condemned."

Regarding your words, your "judgement" and "acquittal" are immediate and ongoing, least of which is the affect they cause in other people that hear you speak.

God wants you to speak a common, more spiritually sensitive, language now. To harmonize with Him and the rest of His loving children. One based on understanding and love. So that, together with others, you may be empowered as a unified and spiritually intelligent congregation. He wishes you to be uplifted by His revelations of knowledge, including those herein about speech, language, the spoken word, and how these can work for you to create your physical realities. These should all serve His Messianic Kingdom, "on earth as it is in Heaven," and leave devil-doers in the dust.

Reverse Speech and the English Language

When I heard the thesis of David John Oates, the man who pioneered the field of "reverse speech," I was intrigued. "The English language and speech played backwards, relays the truth of the soul," he claimed. On national radio he played segments of famous people's speeches, but backwards. Very clearly you could hear completely different messages than expected. For instance, one speech of President Bill Clinton played backwards revealed highly denigrating comments about himself! Another reverse speech assignment I paid David John Oates to perform provided a completely accurate personality assessment of a colleague. Then, he ran one of my lectures and radio interviews in reverse, and gave me my analysis. Indeed, he was completely accurate in deciphering "truth from my soul" of which only I was aware.

So I began to investigate his theory and technology further. Based on this study, and the information relayed in greater detail in *Healing Codes for the Biological Apocalypse*, I must conclude that English is mathematically related, if not derived, from the ancient sacred languages, particularly Hebrew. Unfortunately, it's mathematically, electromagnetically, and spiritually *backwards*!

English, you know, reads from left to right while Hebrew reads from right to left. Why? Ultimately, because of the spiritual warfare directed against the ignorant masses. Scientific research shows the right hemisphere of your brain is functionally related more to spirituality and intuitive instincts than to the earthy desires and rational reasoning processed mostly in your left hemisphere. Brain function relates to language too. When the direction of reading words and articulating them in speech is reversed, as it is when Divine Hebrew is translated into Babylonian English, it literally violates your Spiritual connection and optimal brain function.

The Hebrews, who received God's first covenant, were empowered by their birthright, bloodlines, *and sacred language* to maintain a closer Spiritual connection to God. Subsequently, to control the world, better manipulate and "dumb down" the masses so-to-speak, English was contrived mathematically to confound this spiritual channel. Your electromagnetic link to God was thusly compromised. Your spoken word, upon which Yeshua said you are judged, either reflects this powerful Spiritual connection to God, and thereby your residence in the Holy Kingdom, or it doesn't.

Healing Language in the Holy Kingdom

Ideally, to make God happy, our Father desires His loving children to walk righteously and joyfully "on earth as it is in Heaven." That means, God's Holy Kingdom is available to you right NOW. This implies a modus operandi—a mode of operations—dealing with life as a sublime Spirit of willingness to produce miracles and blessings consistently in your life. You enter into this Holy Kingdom simply by following His laws which are His *Word* relayed in the Bible. When you are living and traveling in this dimension, then your every step is ordered by Him as Proverbs 20:24 and Jeremiah 10:23 attests. Thus, you will be, or are, walking in health, prosperity, joy, and grace according to His covenant which is described in Genesis 26:5 and Matthew 24:45-47. Therefore, His covenant, His desire, is your contract to share a miraculously healthy life in His Kingdom right here and now!

King David, in his prayer to God in Psalms 17:4-5, beautifully summarized this opportunity and Spiritual connection relating to the importance of words, Divinely ordered steps, and subsequent heavenly rewards. He prayed, "You probed my heart, you visited me at night, and you assayed me without finding evil thoughts that should not pass my lips. As for what others do, by words from your lips I have kept myself from the ways of the violent; my steps hold steadily to your paths, my feet do not slip."

Further clarity regarding the power of language, and the speech that flows from your lips, is provided in James 3:2-11 which reads:

> For we all stumble in many ways; if someone does not stumble in what he says, he is a mature man who can bridle his whole body. If we put a bit into a horse's mouth to make it obey us, we control its whole body as well. And think of a ship—although it is huge and is driven by strong winds, yet the pilot can steer it where ever he wants with just a small rudder. So too the tongue is a tiny part of the body, yet it boasts great things. See how a little fire sets a whole forest ablaze! Yes, the tongue is fire, a world of wickedness [or potential goodness in Godly praise and expressing heartfelt love]. The tongue is so placed in our body that it defiles every part of it, setting ablaze the whole of our life . . . With it we bless Adonai, the Father; and with it we curse people, who were made in the image of God. Out of the same mouth come blessing and cursing! Brothers, it isn't right for things to be this way. A spring doesn't send both fresh and bitter water from the same opening, does it?

Briefly summarizing the power of the spoken word and language in your life, Proverbs 18:20-21 says:

> A person's belly will be filled with the fruit of his mouth; with what his lips produce he will be filled. The tongue has power over life and death; those who indulge it must eat its fruit.

So when the English language, and likely other languages as well, were formed, and the direction of reading, sound of the words, and electromagnetics and mathematics of speech was reversed, then the pure unadulterated expression of people's souls became suppressed as well. This profoundly affects you! "The mass of men lead lives of quiet desperation," wrote existentialist poet Henry David Thoreau, mostly because you are spiritually handicapped by the suppressed expression of your

soul through language and speech. Your divine spirit is scream-
ing to be heard, acknowledged, and loved, as you long to celebrate health, happiness, and prosperity through your connection
to God and others. The resolution and restoration is at hand. The
Father, His Son, and their Holy Spirit are working in unison to
rectify this earthy deception, reverse the damage, and celebrate
with you the prophesied thousand years of world peace.

Spiritual Ignorance and God's Language

If you can't get this simple profound truth about your spoken
words creating your life, hell or heaven, then you are not alone.
Especially difficult to comprehend is the electromagnetic matrix
of creative potential accessed by faith and prayer through the
Holy Spirit. This is most critical for miraculous healings.

Yeshua's emissary Sha'ul, better known as Apostle Paul,
advised the Messianic Jewish community about their Spiritual
ignorance in this regard. He discussed connections between
sound, words, and the Spirit of God, in 1 Corinthians 2:6-16. He
wrote:

> Yet there is a wisdom that we are speaking to those who
> are mature enough for it. But it is not the wisdom of
> this world, or of this world's leaders, who are in the
> process of passing away. On the contrary, we are com-
> municating a secret wisdom from God which has been
> hidden until now which, before history began, God had
> decreed would bring us glory. Not one of this world's
> leaders has understood it; because if they had, they
> would not have executed the Lord from whom this
> glory flows. But, as the *Tanakh* says,
>
> **"No eye has seen, no ear has heard**
> **and no one's heart has imaged**
> **all the things that God has prepared**
> **for those who love him."**
>
> It is to us, however, that God has revealed these things.
> How? Through the Spirit. For the Spirit probes all
> things, even the most profound depths of God. For who

knows the inner workings of a person except the
person's own spirit inside him? So too no one knows
the inner workings of God except God's Spirit. Now we
have not received the spirit of the world but the Spirit
of God, so that we might understand the things God has
so freely given us. These are the things we are talking
about when we avoid the manner of speaking that human wisdom would dictate and instead use a manner of
speaking taught by the Spirit, by which we explain
things of the Spirit to people who have the Spirit. Now
the natural man does not receive the things from the
Spirit of God — to him they are nonsense! Moreover,
he is unable to grasp them . . . But the person who has
the Spirit can evaluate everything . . . .

As for me, brothers, I couldn't talk to you as spiritual
people but as worldly people, as babies, so far as experience with the Messiah is concerned. I gave you milk,
not solid food, because you were not yet ready for it.
But you aren't ready for it now either! For you are still
worldly! Isn't it obvious from all the jealousy and quar-
relling among you that you are worldly and living by
merely human standards? . . .

Yeshua's own teachings, and Paul's Divine counsel, therefore, speak of a level of spiritual deprivation that is pandemic.
1 Corinthians 13:11 and 14:1-12 continues:

When I was a child, I spoke like a child,
thought like a child, argued like a child;
now that I have become a man,
I have finished with childish ways. . . .

[K]eep on eagerly seeking the things of the Spirit; and
especially seek to be able to prophesy. For someone
speaking in a tongue is not speaking to people but to
God, because no one can understand, since he is utter-
ing mysteries in the power of the Spirit. But someone
prophesying is speaking to people, edifying, encouraging, and comforting them. A person speaking in a
tongue does edify himself, but a person prophesying

edifies the congregation. I wish you would all speak in tongues, but even more I wish you would all prophesy. The person who prophesies is greater than the person who speaks in tongues, unless someone gives an interpretation, so that the congregation can be edified.

Brothers, suppose I come to you now speaking in tongues. How can I be of benefit to you unless I bring you some revelation or knowledge or prophecy or teaching? Even with lifeless musical instruments, such as a flute or a harp, how will anyone recognize the melody if one note can't be distinguished from another? And if the bugle gives an unclear sound, who will get ready for battle? It's the same with you: how will anyone know what you are saying unless you use your tongue to produce intelligible speech? You will be talking to the air!

There are undoubtedly all kinds of sounds in the world, and none is altogether meaningless; but if I don't know what a person's sounds mean, I will be a foreigner to the speaker and the speaker will be a foreigner to me. Likewise with you: since you eagerly seek the things of the Spirit, seek especially what will help in edifying [defined as "to instruct or improve in spiritual knowledge"] the congregation."

This is precisely what I intend to convey with this chapter— revelations about the creative power behind language, words, and Spirit—an edification of the congregation and uplifting of the Church. The meaning of God's special sounds, as we shared in *Healing Codes for the Biological Apocalypse,* imparts an understanding of your power to heal your life using the sounds of your spoken words. Your lips are, therefore, electromagnetic creative instruments. Indeed, this is vitally important information for personal and world health. Using this knowledge the manipulated masses can be freed from their ignorance.

Speech, tones, sounds, music, and the vibratory essence of Spirit, are all mathematics and frequencies based. These are all vital areas of growing scientific knowledge during this revolutionary period in human history. Spiritual evolution *is* the Divine focus of this book, and the musical harmonic force behind everything! Spiritually mature people, empowered to act on this wisdom, and thus be healed and whole, hold the power to rectify the primary problem that has plagued humanity since the "Tower of Babel."

Simply speaking, using God's Babylonian method of controlling people by introducing dialects, society was later manipulated by a few evil men who further divided the "sheeple" from each other, and from God, by dispensing foreign languages and contaminated tongues. Thereafter, humanity largely ceased speaking Spiritually uplifting syllables. You were thus, at least partly, cut off from the free flow of Divine love God endlessly bestows. To recapture what was lost, you simply need to speak God's language once again. Have your lips move to express truth, love, faith, praise, and harmony.

More on Bioelectrics and Healing:
The Suppressed Work of Royal R. Rife

Like healing words that express electromagnetic frequencies, so too can machines produce frequencies of sound, light, and colors that heal.

In the 1940s, based largely on the brilliant work of Nikola Tesla, Royal Raymond Rife became the first to microscopically confirm the theory that infectious microbes can change form. Using innovative electromagnetic light refraction techniques and crystal technologies in his splendid microscopes, Rife observed bacteria transform into viruses and fungi, and sometimes, depending on the "terrain," back again.

Rife became America's, if not the world's leading microscopist. In fact, his work might have changed the face of modern medicine were it not for the ruthless persecution he received at the hands of the "medical mafia"—the Rockefeller-directed medical–industrial complex. His story is best told in *The Cancer Cure That Worked!* by Barry Lynes. It included a description of

Rife's extraordinary microscope. Detailed in the *Journal of the Franklin Institute* (Vol. 237, No. 2, 1944), the Rife Universal Microscope had a 31,000 diameter resolution, weighed 200 pounds, stood two feet high, and consisted of 5,682 parts. It used natural light frequencies dispersed by glass or crystal prisms, rather than acid stains or electronic beams, to view *live* objects in extraordinary detail. For instance, one microscope was even able to measure "crystal angles" at the cancer virus protein level.

Rife observed the pleomorphic transformation of viruses in cancerous tissues. He recorded them becoming fungi. Then, he planted these fungi in a plant-based medium. Spontaneously, a bacteria, typically found in the human intestine, developed. He repeated the study with the same results several hundred times. Later, he used this knowledge to apply resonant frequencies to cure these infections as well as reverse certain cancers.

Also, based largely on Nikola Tesla's studies in frequency science, Royal Rife developed his electromagnetic frequency-generating healing devices. He studied these for years. He began by identifying radio frequencies that could irradiate and kill tubercle bacilli—the bacteria associated with tuberculosis. Using trial and error, he finally succeeded in killing the germ, but the guinea pigs he used for the experiment died of "toxic poisoning."

Rife reasoned that viruses within the bacteria, that were not destroyed by the resonant frequency, had been released when the bacilli broke apart. To study the viruses, however, he needed to enhance his microscopic resolution. To do this, he conceived of a "method of staining the virus with light." Again the idea used resonant frequencies of light that he knew were found inherent in, and specific to, every microorganism. Rife demonstrated that light, rather than deadly chemicals, could be used to "stain" the subjects being studied, and thus observed them in their natural living condition.

By the end of his research, Rife had developed an entire book listing the specific frequencies associated with virtually every disease and every microbe, and the electromagnetic frequencies required to treat them. This work naturally captured the attention of numerous members of the scientific, medical, *and* intelligence communities.

Scientists and physicians from around the world hailed Rife's work and sojourned to observe for themselves its legitimacy. His list of respected colleagues and observers included: Dr. Edward C. Rosenow of the Mayo Clinic; Dr. Milbank Johnson, a member of the board of directors at California's Pasadena Hospital, and Dr. Arthur I. Kendall, Director of Medical Research at Northwestern University Medical School. Newspapers heralded Rife's progress. His favorable notoriety seemed so infectious that his enemies were moved to act.

Morris Fishbein, a Rockefeller puppet at the helm of the American Medical Association when the U.S. Supreme Court found the organization guilty of antitrust violations during the late 1930s and early 1940s, persecuted Rife and personally organized an attack against him. Fishbein learned of Rife's successful resonant frequency method of treating cancer. He then approached Rife with a "buy in" offer that the inventor refused. Fishbein then brought suit against Rife's company for "practicing medicine without a license."

Unfortunately, Rife's timing couldn't have been worse. He began researching frequency microscopy and electromagnetics for healing in the early 1920s—virtually the same time the Rockefeller family created the cancer industry and gained control over American medicine. Rife's life's work was said to be a simple, safe, and inexpensive answer to cancer. The Rockefellers preferred a costly and risky pharmaceutical approach.

Other Research in Vibrational Medicine and "Bio-Spiritual Warfare"

In addition to the works of Chladni, Jenny, Tesla and Rife etc., other scientists have proven the critical biological impact of electromagnetics and frequency vibrations. They are all referenced in, *Healing Codes for the Biological Apocalypse.*

In 1923, for instance, a Russian anatomy professor, Dr. A. G. Gurvich, advanced a theory that ultraviolet light was essential to one of life's greatest mysteries—cell division. He had pointed the root tip of a growing onion toward the side of a second proliferating onion root. He noticed that the cells of the latter in the area of the root tip divided much faster. He theorized that ultraviolet light, or some other electromagnetic "mitogenetic radiation," was likely responsible for the biological change later called the "Gurvich Effect."

During the following decade teams of mostly German and Russian scientists attempted to confirm the "Gurvich Effect" without success. After more than 500 research papers were published in this field of study, the subject was dropped. Then it was resurrected in the 1950s with the development of the photon-counter photomultiplier. This technology, aided by cryogenic techniques, enabled photodetectors to be cooled to very low temperatures, and allowed researchers to confirm the "Gurvich Effect"—the effect of mitogenetic radiation on cells.

Central to "bio-spiritual warfare," by 1974, Dr. V.F. Kaznachayev and his associates showed that *ultraviolet light frequencies could transmit viral induced infections between cell cultures.* These researchers arranged "pairs of sealed glass tubes containing healthy cell cultures end to end separated only by a sheet of quartz." After inoculating one culture with a deadly virus, the investigators were surprised to learn the adjacent sterile culture had also become ill.

When they duplicated the experiment with the quartz sheet removed, the sterile culture adjacent to the infected one remained unaffected. The glass tubes alone could not transmit the electromagnetic frequencies required to communicate the disease. In other words, special disease frequencies were *trans-*

mitted by the quartz crystal and these alone were sufficient to infect the sterile cell cultures!

After repeatedly reproducing these results, the Russian team surmised that when the infected cells in culture died, they emitted UV light which was transmitted through the quartz to the adjacent cell cultures. These electromagnetic frequency transmissions then induced, like progressive crystal growth, progressive cell death in the initially healthy cultures.

Kaznachayev's team also showed that with the introduction of a virus into cell cultures, a change in the photon emissions of the cells was seen even before cell degeneration and death occurred.

Then, as the cell cultures died, they were observed to change their UV frequency radiations again. This suggested to Dr. Kaznachayev and his colleagues, that disease processes could possibly be altered by determining the dying cell frequency emissions and intercepting or neutralizing them before they had a chance to kill adjacent cells or tissues within their energy field. Additional support for this theory came from the observation that yeast cell reproduction could be slowed using specific UV light frequencies.

Given these observations, they concluded, "We feel we may then learn to affect healing by altering the photon flux before it contaminates neighboring systems."

Clearly, these findings could have profound implications on treating and preventing a variety of diseases, if research in this field was not suppressed. As you will soon learn, destructive uses of this knowledge takes government precedence.

In 1974, the esteemed scientific journal *Biochemistry Biophysics Research Communication* published a study by two Western scientists who detected a "weak chemiluminescence" coming from yeast UV frequency emissions.

Ultra-weak UV emissions and visible light in the range of 200-800 nanometers have also been seen coming from a variety of organisms and cells during mitosis. *These radiation frequencies were found associated with cellular DNA. Stored photon energy is apparently associated with the nucleic acids, that is the nucleotides, that comprise the genetic double helix.* Scientists proposed this model might best explain a wide array of biological observations.

As mentioned, estimates indicate *only 0.1-2 percent of DNA functions as genetic material. The vast majority of the helical strand not involved in coding for protein synthesis is believed to function electromagnetically.* The six-sided crystal clustered water molecules structurally supporting the nucleotide strands, and protein enzymes, apparently play a primary role in regulating every aspect of cellular metabolism. Additional evidence for this comes from the fact that when cells die, they release stored photons as "coherent, monochromatic, energy sources with properties similar to laser light. . . . UV radiation from a laser has been shown to stimulate DNA synthesis and change the permeability of cell membranes."

Dr. Schjelderup, a Norwegian doctor has suggested that viruses might emit lethal electromagnetic (EM) radiations, and thus kill cells in culture. He added that viral infections might thereby transmit disease by specific frequency emissions besides physical or genetic contact.

In the realm of "bio-spiritual warfare" once again, much experimental evidence has accumulated to support the notion that a spectrum of EM fields cause illness. In most cases, very weak signals were found to have the greatest effects whereas strong signals produced none at all. Therefore, the toxic effects of frequency vibrations are most commonly associated with only very tiny specific EM amplitudes and wave frequencies. In today's world, you can't escape the myriad electromagnetic frequency fields and vibrations that add to natural background radiation and environmental pollution. These can profoundly impact your health.

Without going into great detail, the use of extremely high powered electromagnetic energy transmitters, documented on a U.S. Government website called Project HAARP, and its European counterpart, Project EISCAT, as discussed in great detail in *Healing Codes for the Biological Apocalypse*, presents great and grave risks to humanity. These "ionospheric heating" centers direct electromagnetic frequency signals toward the ionosphere, the highest level of the atmosphere. The signals bounce back and heat things up, like small areas of the South Pacific. You've heard of El Niño. HAARP's frequency emissions and ionospheric scatter-back are the likeliest cause of El Niño and the related changes in weather patterns and the jet stream.

It is beyond the scope of this book to defend this assertion. It's sufficient to warn you here that the bioelectric technologies that U.S. Government agencies have been suppressing, are being used to manipulate weather, and worse, in keeping with the *Report From Iron Mountain* that I discuss at length in *Healing Codes for the Biological Apocalypse*. At the end of this work you will realize that no matter how you prepare for the plagues, famine, pestilence, and "natural" disasters prophesied in the Bible, given this new advanced level of "bio-spiritual warfare," you are lost without God's protective hand over your life.

This simply leaves you to implement the advice provided in Ephesians 6:15-19 where it is written:

> Take up the shield of faith, with which you can extinguish all the flaming arrows of the evil one. Take the helmet of salvation and the sword of the Spirit, which is the work of God. And pray in the Spirit on all occasions with all kinds of prayers and requests. . . . Pray also for me, that whenever I open my mouth, words may be given me so that I will fearlessly make known the mystery of the gospel, for which I am an ambassador in chains. Pray that I may declare it fearlessly, as I should.

As for you, be "wise as a serpent and as gentle as a dove." Be aware of what the enemy, the Adversary, is up to, and fear not if you partake in the glory of God. As Psalms 91 prophesies, "A thousand may fall at your side, ten thousand at your right hand, but [evil] will not come near you" if you have faith in the Lord and abide by His laws.

Chapter 7.
Healing Words

"Go . . . to the lost sheep of the house of Isra'el.
As you go, proclaim, 'The Kingdom of Heaven is near,'
heal the sick, raise the dead,
cleanse those afflicted with plagues, expel the demons. . .
Pay attention!
I am sending you out like sheep among wolves,
so be as prudent as snakes and as harmless as doves. . . .
For it will not be just you speaking, but the Spirit of your
heavenly Father speaking through you."

Yeshua speaking in Matthew 10:6-20,
The Complete Jewish Bible

Obviously, no matter how often, or great, the presence of evil comes, God's good always prevails. It has been, and always will be, that way. In this chapter, I will examine the scriptural words for personal and world healing. In earlier chapters, the latest scientific advances related to spiritual healing were considered with occasional reference to relevant Bible verses. In this chapter, I will focus on the scriptures you need to integrate and apply in your life to actualize miraculous healings while walking in the "Kingdom of Heaven" here on earth. *Here* I will relay God's words for Divine personal and world healing. Contrary to popular belief, God wants you healed, living among healthy people, and enjoying a peaceful planet. Here you will examine His scriptural covenant, his contract with you, for health, healing, prosperity, and the joy-filled achievement of your beneficent destiny.

In this chapter you will consider six major areas of your life and the related Bible verses regarding: 1) why God wants you to be healed and live in health and prosperity; 2) why trust in your relationship with God is imperative if you intend to miraculously heal every aspect of your life; 3) how and why words from your lips become powerful creative forces for health and healing; 4) how and why you should prepare for miraculous healings, and fully expect them to come about; 5) why heartfelt love is a prerequisite for maximum anointing with God's Divine power that you can then use to help others heal through the Holy Spirit; and 6) why forgiveness of sin, your own and other's, is required to live your life in freedom and peace, as well as health and prosperity.

God's Healing Covenant

The quote introducing this chapter is your guarantee and reminder that God is ready, willing, and able to produce miraculous healings for you. That is, if you simply follow His Divine loving laws. Even raising the dead is not an impossibility when you are empowered by His redeeming Spirit. You too can be a miracle worker, a supernaturally inspired vessel through which His Divine energy flows to "heal the sick, raise the dead, cleanse those afflicted [and] expel demons."

Now God lays out His covenant, his contract, with you to perform all the above in no uncertain terms. His words and agreements are meticulously articulated in the Bible. Misinterpretations from the purely human perspective, often block even God-loving Bible-reading people from experiencing the truth, and mustering the faith in Him and His word required to fulfill his covenant, and thereby reap the rewards from His contractual agreements.

"Listen carefully to me, and you will eat well, you will enjoy the fat of the land," God urges and offers in Isaiah 55:1-3. "Open your ears, and come to me; listen well and you will live—I will make an *everlasting covenant* with you, the grace I assured. . ."

Notice He prescribes *listening*, opening your ears to the sounds of His words. As I explained in the previous chapter, the sound of His words deliver spiritually uplifting syllables— Divine electromagnetic and bioacoustic force fields designed to raise you up into His light and perfect health.

Like all loving parents who wish to play with their children as they grow, He too wishes to empower you to listen and co-create, according to His "everlasting covenant," supernatural health, vitality, joy, and prosperity.

This should not be new to you. This truth has been around for awhile. In Exodus 23:22-26, Moses bade his followers, "If you listen to what He says, and do everything I tell you, then I will be an enemy to your enemies and a foe to your foes . . . You are to serve Adonai, your God; and he will bless your food and water. I will take sickness away from among you. . . . your women will not be barren, and you will live out the full span of your lives."

From at least the time of Abraham, God heralded His contract for human blessings. "I will make your descendants as numerous as the stars in the sky," God told Abraham. "I will give all these lands to your descendants, and by your descendants all the nations of the earth will bless *themselves*. All of this is because Abraham heeded what I said and did what I told him to do—he followed my commandments, my regulations, and my teachings." (See Genesis 26:4-5.)

Notice even God tells you His blessings come through *you*. That is, by following His laws, you immediately enter into the glorious Kingdom of Heaven wherein you should expect ongoing miraculous blessings. Following this prescription, for instance, Abraham's son Isaac "planted crops in the land and reaped . . . a hundred times as much as he had sowed. God had blessed him." These supernatural results, and ongoing miracles like it, are only possible by following His laws; and, thereby, manifesting His Kingdom "on earth as it is in Heaven" as Yeshua explained in Matthew 6:10.

The Bible also cautions those who have recently moved into His Heavenly Kingdom against being evicted. "Eviction notices" rapidly arrive as soon as your ego begins to believe in conceit that you, in all your greatness, inscribed yourself into the Father's favor. You may think to yourself, "My own power and the strength of my own hand have gotten me this" wealth and health. This is a trap cautioned against in Deuteronomy 8:17 wherein God warns, "No, you are to remember Adonai your God, because *it is He who is giving you the power to get wealth, in order to confirm His covenant*, which He swore to your ancestors, as is happening even today."

God keeps His word. He made a covenant—a contract—with Abraham which continues to this very day. "He swore it to your ancestors!" He is, therefore, bound by His word, glory, and goal to see His children, healthy, whole, and uplifted in His Holy Spirit. To the extent that any of His children continue a sinful existence, God, who battles the Adversary for a place in your heart, is saddened. "Hear oh Israel, the Lord our God, the Lord is One." In His Holy Spirit, we are all one with God and each other. Anyone who violates the faith, trust, and spirit—energy—of this binding contract, degrades our unity a bit. God doesn't want to lose even an inch to Satan. This is the reason He wishes you to have faith in Him and His commandments. With your faith and trust comes His glory—His miraculous blessings, including healings. Are you ready for them? "Trust and ye shall receive."

Satan versus God

Many people believe that God wills disease, hardship, and premature death. Absolutely not! God wills health, healing, joy, and prosperity. Knowledge of this comes from the book of Job.

God pulled his protective hand from Job in order to teach him and Satan a lesson. My daughter and I had a very similar lesson taught to us.

One day, a colleague whom I greatly respect, challenged me with his position that Satan, the great Adversary, was not really a spiritual being. It is merely a misleading label, he argued, a manipulative tool of religion covering the greater likelihood that "God is all there is, . . . and you cause your own strife by losing faith and violating God's laws." His premise, he said, was "supported by scripture," including a lack of Satan's specific definition in his Concordance.

Desiring for God to show me the truth in His word about this, I prayed, "God, show me the truth about your relationship to Satan." Then I opened the Bible. I found fifteen references to "Satan" and five to the "Adversary." I read these verses. Then I read "The Wisdom of Solomon" in the Apocrypha that dealt with this specific issue—the battle between good versus evil, God versus Satan. I was ninety-nine percent sure that my colleague was completely off base—totally wrong, but there remained that one percent of doubt.

The next day I flew to Atlanta, with my seven-year-old daughter, to give a lecture and then take a well deserved vacation—"just Daddy and his little girl." During our flight, while tutoring Alena in math, I became extremely frustrated. I found that she really wasn't paying attention. I knew that she had the wherewithal to do this homework assignment, but it seemed as though she just wasn't receiving my simple explanations and instructions.

That night, Dr. John Donofrio, the meeting director, picked us up from the airport. Accompanied by two colleagues who took our luggage in their car because John's trunk was filled to capacity with seminar manuals, we all drove off to our hotel. "Make sure your seatbelts are fastened. Especially Alena's," he cautioned. "We don't want any harm coming to you." I reached back from the passenger seat to secure Alena's seatbelt, and then fastened my own.

Minutes later, on the interstate doing about 60 m.p.h., as I was enthusiastically sharing with the good Christian doctor my most recent revelations about the power and electrodynamics of prayer, a dreadful accident began. A tractor trailer truck driving on our right failed to see us in his "blindspot." He ventured into our lane and hit the front right quarter of our vehicle. That pushed John, at the wheel, into a 60 m.p.h. head spin left as he lost control of the car.

At this point, all I could do was pray. I called loudly, strongly, and repeatedly to God for his angelic protection. Realizing we had numerous vehicles behind us, all going at high speeds, I focused intently on the Lord, and repeatedly pleaded for His Divine intervention and protection.

As we swerved left entering the "high speed" lane, another eighteen wheeler was about to pass. Obviously unable to avoid the collision, John and I watched, from what felt like a bubble, as this tractor trailer truck smashed through the left front of our car sending the front end assembly flying forward along the highway. This sent our car suddenly spinning right.

At this point, while continuing to plead prayerfully to God, my concern shifted to my sweet little angel—Alena—who by now realized something dreadful was happening. She had never been in an accident before. As I reached back to comfort her, our vehicle still spinning right, I saw out of the corner of my eye another eighteen wheeler about to strike the rear of our car. A direct hit might kill her, I realized. Grabbing her shoulder was all I could do to brace her against the impending impact. The Mack truck struck a powerful blow to the trunk. The entire trunk caved in with the seminar manuals acting as a cushion for Alena's protection. Now we began spinning left once again, but came to a stop in the middle of the highway. As I looked back, I suddenly realized the accident was over. All traffic in back of us had stopped. My prayers to God were answered.

Chanting praises to God in glorious thanks I exited the totally demolished rental car. I reached in to pick Alena up from the back seat, then carried her to the side of the highway realizing that those who came running to help us had all witnessed a miracle. John, also unharmed, followed closely behind me.

Can you imagine one midsize car, being struck at high speed not once, not twice, but three times by three eighteen wheelers, and all three passengers walking out virtually unscratched?

About an hour later in our hotel room, as I prepared a hot bath to steady our nerves, Alena said that her left ear hurt. The only injury any of us sustained was this—the tip of Alena's left ear had been mildly bruised by its impact against the door when the third truck hit us.

"Isn't that interesting," I thought, as I reflected on my frustrating attempt to have her *listen and receive* my math instructions earlier that day. "The left side of her body, in wholistic medicine, represents the receptive side. She could hear me, but she wasn't *receiving* my instructions. God's protective hand was removed only from this tiny part of Alena's body so that, in His great mercy, she would learn the lesson to *'listen and receive.'*"

Then it dawned on me that the accident was an answer to my prayer as well. I had asked God to "show me your relationship with Satan." As in the story of Job, God pulled His protective hand away from the very tip of my loved one's ear to teach me that, indeed, he is the Great Protector, who can choose to allow Satan to do his dirty work. The Masterful control demonstrated to deliver this lesson through a most miraculous event is truly a signature work by God.

Satan too was taught a lesson that day. As a spiritual entity, he is impotent in comparison to the Lord. Now I get to tell the world about this relationship.

Relationships Based on Trust

Can you imagine any relationship lasting without faith and trust? Consider a marriage between partners who don't trust each other. How about business partners who share little or no faith in their contract? Not very hopeful pictures, are they? That's why God simply demands trust in your relationship with Him. Once you have that, then everything else falls into place, including your social and marital relationships. As Yeshua advises in Matthew 6:33, "But seek first His Kingdom and his Righteousness, and all these things will be given to you as well."

Allow me to digress for a few paragraphs to relay another true story with relevance to the topic of functional relationships.

Not long before I sold my dental practice in 1993 for a career in investigative journalism and public speaking, a patient, still very much in love with her husband, shared how he was abusing her. Not physically, but mentally and emotionally as is all too common. In fact, as I reflected on my own relationship with my loving wife, I pleaded guilty to the same offense.

Why did God create marriages to bring out the best, as well as worst, in people? The answer lies in the same age old battle between good and evil, God versus Satan. This rages insidiously within spouses. There is a spiritual and biblical perspective on this dynamic that you might want to consider, along with some practical recommendations to turn the "madness" you might be experiencing in your marriage, your partnership(s), and your covenant/contract with God, into opportunities for lifelong learning, love, and spiritual enrichment.

In the Book of Genesis, God spoke the Universe into existence in six days, breathed the breath of life into Adam's nostrils, then took from him a rib to make his mate, Eve. Eve was to provide service and inspiration to Adam forever.

Formed in their Father's image, along with the power God gave Adam and Eve to co-create, came the power for them to destroy. Then came their great fall from grace. As long as Adam and Eve followed God's commandments, they stayed blessed within a nurturing matrix of His electromagnetic Spirit. Their Godly image and essence remained intact as long as they followed His loving rules. Temptation, however, persuaded them to transgress His laws. They thus violated His faith and trust, the basis of all relationships, partnerships, and especially marriages. Adam and Eve's Divine, fully-empowered relationship with their Father was abruptly compromised that day. They suddenly knew and felt fear. With their Divine self-images grossly tarnished, they covered their reproductive parts. This physical dressing symbolically covered their guilt. Thus began humanity's great fall from Godkind to mankind.

Guilt, Selfishness, or Pride, Not God, Always Comes Before the Fall

Guilt is essentially fear associated with knowing, in your heart, that you have done something wrong in the past and may be called upon to pay for your transgression sometime in the future.

When Adam, led by Eve and temptation, rather than God, stepped "off the mark" and into the realm of feasting on forbidden fruit, the image of God that the Father had projected with faith through His lips into His children's hearts and souls was shattered along with their positive self-images. They suddenly felt ashamed and guilty. Not ashamed of the perfect reflection of God that they were, but ashamed of the naked disrespectful creations they had become by falling for a serpent's deception, and committing their indiscretions. Their fall, and the shattering of their positive self-images, involved pain, shame, guilt, loss, and a perceived threat to survival. It pained them to realize they had violated God's faith, jeopardized his trust, and lost a large measure of His gracious sustenance. Adam was, after all, required thereafter to work ceaselessly for his food whereas before God gave it to him freely.

It is said that selfishness and pride always comes before the fall. In Adam's case, he blamed Eve for his sin rather than taking responsibility for violating his covenant with God. In the case of their children, Cain and Abel, the former murdered the later due to jealousy and anger. God then sentenced Cain to a life of hardship.

As in the days of Adam and Eve, with their fall from grace, so it is today with people who step out of the nurturing Spirit of God's love, and into the realm of deception and strife.

People form all sorts of negative beliefs, attitudes, and behaviors by adulthood. These influence behavior and affect relationships too often for the worse. Mature adults often recognize their shortcomings. In moments of self reflection they glimpse back to the way their parents molded them into this type of abusive behavior. Much of it boils down to the classic "monkey see, monkey do" activity. Self and socially destructive behaviors get passed on generation to generation, to the detriment of everyone, including God. And he's not very happy about it. For, in this way, his children take on negative self-images that undermine their self-esteem. Have you become a mere shadow of the person God intended you to be? Do you often express yourself in anger, jealously, resentment, or aggression in place of tolerance, empathy, love, and affection?

Marriages and Marriage Contracts

Now God, in all His great mercy, understands this is part of the fallen human condition. To help, He sends us counselors and therapists who see through our myriad shortcomings, and reflect them back to us in an effort to help extinguish the neurosis and free us, once again, to live healthier, more whole, and less troubled lives. This is the unofficial practical definition of a spouse!

In fact, what married couples do best, intentionally or not, is mirror one another's best, *and worst,* traits. Emphasis most commonly gets placed on the worst. That, by itself, can become a stumbling block to pleasant marital relations. In fact, it is a rare, strongly loving, and most commonly female, person who most ably transcends these emotionally charged pitfalls, and the destructive dynamics they generate. The softer sex, generally speaking, nurtures her mate through the required spiritual healing process toward complete recovery.

What is being recovered, in truth, is the kind of person God intended; which is "Godkind" evolved from mankind through His love emanating through an open human heart. Likewise, the best facilitator for this transformation and transcendence, most ably maintains an open loving heart.

In fact, women are often more adept at maintaining an open heart, and reflecting their husband's messes—that is, who they are not—because of the extra Divinity in females. The Hebrew word for man is "ish," and woman is "ish*ah*." So women, according to the derivation of the word, as told in the Book of Genesis, are men with an extra measure of God's grace and molding. It's like second generation computers. Everyone knows they function better, have less glitches, and usually have more memory! It is widely recognized that women are, generally speaking, more intuitive and sensitive, while men are generally more rational and aggressive. So it's not surprising that women can more adeptly intuit lovingly, and with open hearts, their mate's barriers to optimal divinity.

With faith and trust in their marriage, and in their spouse, couples can honestly discuss issues that cause strife in their relationships, heal and transcend these, then move on to co-create life with God in service to everyone.

Now isn't that the way marriages, and life, should be? Co-creative and uplifting in every way? God certainly thinks so.

He's working overtime to help create just that. That's why He asked me to write this book. God wants you healthy and whole to reflect a larger part of Him. He longs to express Himself more fully including His immense love for you and humanity. He wants more players on the field instead of in the bleachers. Rather than getting drunk on booze, He prefers you get intoxicated on His love. Of course, the best place to begin is at home with your spouse. Again, "on earth as it is in Heaven." God created the sanctity of marriage, and its contract, to reflect His covenant of grace, forgiveness, and love. Simply keep the vows with both your spouse and God, and He will prosper and heal you.

Trust in God's Desire to Heal His Bride: A Great Victory

The following story, and prophecy being fulfilled, is an example of the power of faithful/trusting marriages between spouses, and between God and His "bride." On the eve of the twentieth anniversary of her successful "Healing School," Gloria Copeland, wife of the famous charismatic minister, and television evangelist, Kenneth Copeland, relayed the following prophecy to her audience. She had received this message first from God, and then through her husband in 1979. After successfully completing her first "healing school," she felt intimidated to continue teaching. Then, while praying on her front porch in Lakeland, Florida, the Lord came to her and said, "Gloria, I want you to teach healing at *every* meeting [from now on] because I want my people well."

A bit overwhelmed about this ongoing healing assignment Gloria told Kenneth about what the Lord said. She asked her husband to pray on it for further clarification. He did, and God gave Kenneth the following message that he quickly relayed to Gloria:

"You've wondered why the [Holy] manifestation has not come on to [you and carried you to] the peaks of . . . this ministry as you know it should. It is because you have been laying back."

Gloria admitted she probably had been "laying back," resting on her laurels, a bit.

Kenneth than said to Gloria, "You've always been part of this ministry. For the Lord said to me in 1967, 'She's precious to me. I've given her to you. She is unto you what temper is to steel.'

"So that needs to come to pass," Kenneth Copeland continued. "In this [first 'healing school'] meeting, as you [Gloria] obeyed God, and took your place, and delivered the message that God told you to deliver, then both parts of the unit [—the marriage between Kenneth and Gloria—] were in full function. That's when it will work most. When you and I together deliver the Word, and the Word will go, and the Word [God] will hear it, and it will work. 'And it shall be as you've desired and prayed,' saithe the Lord. And they will even say, 'In Jesus [they were all healed].'"

Gloria continued, "I believe in that for us today. That every person gets their deliverance from healing!"

A few months later, Kenneth delivered another message from God to Gloria regarding her upcoming "healing schools."

"I want my people well," God said. "I want my people well. I have a job to do that is so vast and so large in its scope that sick people will not be able to carry it out. . . . I want my people well! I have desired for my people to walk in health. I have desired for my people to know *how* to walk in health, regardless of what ministry [they attend]. I want my people to know how to take my Word, and stand on my Word, and *receive my healing power*. And know that *I am Lord*. I want my people to walk with me in health and in life, and know the good things that I have prepared for them. I have set a table before you in the presence of your enemies. You shall not be an orphan group. You shall not go hungry. You shall not be in want. For I am the God provider. I am the Lord God that heals you. I want my people well.

"When you hear someone say that I desire one to be sick," God continued, "you may know, and you may remember this, you may have My voice rise up on the inside of you that will say, 'That is not true! I want my people well!'"

Gloria commented, "When I hear things like that . . . When I hear someone say that God makes you sick to try to teach you something, that's what comes up. [God's voice saying,] 'That is not true! I want my people well!'"

"I have a desire in me," said the Lord. "And my desire is to come unto you. My desire is to get you with me. Not only in me, but *with* me [as the 'bride' in marriage]. . . .

"That means putting Him first," Gloria continued. "He can't get with us when we're wrong, as far as getting His full support [is concerned]. We have to get with Him because He's right. [His laws are just.] We have to change our way of thinking. We have to seek God, and seek the wisdom of God, and be quick to change when we see what He says about things."

"My desire is to get you with me," God repeatedly urged. "Not only *in* me, but *with* me. I desire to see my people doing what I bid them to do, and hurry up. Hurry up! Get this revival completed. Get it finished. Cause the resurrection to come. Then move into the Millennial Reign. I have a desire for this," said the Lord. "My desire is to have my people grow and come to the knowledge of the truth, and understand my words, and understand my ways, and understand my things."

"In fact," Gloria clarified, "since the old covenant, He has always wanted to be understood; for his people to understand His ways. If His family doesn't understand Him and His ways, then they won't walk with Him; they won't seek Him; they can't obey Him, and so He can't manifest Himself [to them.] So here's God's desire. And I feel this is His heart's desire. I can feel that in my heart. 'My desire is to have my people grow, and come to the knowledge of the truth, and understand my words, and understand my ways, and understand my things,' saithe the Lord.

"The way *we* shall do this is for my people to get on *my* Word and be well, and be strong,'" God added, "'All doing their part. All pulling together. And each effect, of every cell in the body doing the work that I've called it to do, edifying the body of Christ in itself in love, and rising to the occasion. Rising to face the enemy. Rising up into a mighty blanket of the Word of God throughout this nation, and throughout the whole world. *I will have my people well!*'" God declared.

So His instruction to Gloria and Kenneth Copeland twenty years earlier was, "Continue this 'healing school' at every morning service until I return, and it will come to pass!"

Victoriously, in 1998, after twenty years of seeing tens of thousands of people miraculously healed, and healing ministries spreading throughout the world, many supported by their efforts, a friend of Kenneth and Gloria Copeland, Pastor Calwell, delivered a prophesy regarding the glory they were witnessing, and that will continue to manifest in the years ahead.

"You have turned a new page," God told Pastor Calwell. "Satan came against you, but you have stood strong and steady. This is a new day of victory. You will begin to see victory in everything you do. The things that have been hard, will become easy. The things that you have been praying for are yours. *Now* is the time to declare victory! Declare victory in your family. Declare victory in your body. Declare victory in your life; in your church. Claim the victory! Claim it everywhere you go, for I have given victory to you. Claim it over every department . . . over all your staff. It is the Spirit of victory that has come over you. Do not take it lightly. Do not take it lightly. Do not take it lightly! . . . Stand fast in the victory, and refuse to have anything less than victory. For there are things that you have prayed for, and forgotten about, that will manifest in victory. Things in your life will be restored to great liberty and victory. You will jump, and sing, and shout as you watch these things come to pass before your eyes. It will not be by your mind, but by my Spirit. You will see it, and witness it, because it will be in your house."

So it has come to pass for many with eyes to read God's word, see His works, and hear His calls. Perhaps this is your destiny too.

Seeking God For Your Victory Over Afflictions

In *The Complete Jewish Bible* (Exodus 15:26), God relayed to Moses His commitment to keeping even His bellyaching people healthy. After traveling in the hot desert for three days without water, God produced a miracle by turning a contaminated well pure for consumption. After saving the Jewish people's water thusly, The Lord told Moses: "If you listen intently to the voice [the scriptural Word] of Adonai, your God, do what He considers right, pay attention to his mitzvot [commandments] and observe His laws, I will not afflict you with any of the diseases I brought on the Egyptians; because I am Adonai your healer."

A friend of mine with a "genetic abnormality" recently called me in a spiritual crisis. A crusader for social justice and public health, he expressed remorse over his lack of political progress with his cause. I told him that I believed his problems stemmed more from spiritual than political blocks; that the power and glory of God was available to him to not only heal the sick, but to "order" his steps, as those of a "righteous man," if he would only observe God's laws and listen for the Lord's voice.

In response, my friend questioned me begrudgingly, "You mean to say that I'm to blame for both my illness and lack of success just because I don't have enough faith in God?"

"I said nothing about blame, did I?" I replied. "You made up that condemnation entirely on your own. But the fact is if you developed your faith, began consulting His word, and followed His laws, you wouldn't need to worry about either your genetic problem, or your political one, because God will handle all of your problems if you would only let Him."

"How is it possible God could 'handle' my genetic problem?" he asked sarcastically. "That's like making blind people see."

"That's precisely how powerful He is. The Bible is full of examples wherein Jesus and the Apostles helped many blind people see by restoring or exercising their faith in God. I just spent the weekend at John G. Lake's 'Healing Rooms' in Spokane, Washington. That's precisely the kind of miracles they witness there. You just need to read the Bible! Just sit down, pray to God, ask Him to show you where in the Bible you need to begin to get reacquainted with His power and glory. Then start heeding His Word, developing your faith and trust in Him, and then give your "insurmountable" problems over to Him and see how easily He handles them. As God said in 2 Kings 20:5, for those who follow Him, 'I have heard your prayer and seen your tears, and I will heal you.'"

My friend just would not get it. He willed to be right, and remain victimized. After all the years of begrudged battling, he was heavily invested in doing it his way rather than God's way. That left me sad, as God Himself feels the loss of His children.

He might have greatly benefited had he read 2 Chronicles 7:13-14. Here God counseled King Solomon, David's son, after he had built God's temple. The Lord "appeared to Solomon by night, and said to him, 'I have heard your prayer . . . If I shut up the sky so that there is no rain; or if I order locusts to devour the land; or if I send an epidemic of sickness among my people; then, if my people, who bear my name, will humble themselves, pray, seek my face and turn from their evil ways, I will hear from heaven, forgive their sin and heal their land.'" Clearly, this is what I had desired and prescribed for my friend.

I firmly believe that trust in God, as said in the Bible, is the only thing required for miraculous progress and healings. This is the success formula prescribed in this chapter. If you only make the smallest sincere commitment to seeking God for your progress or healing, or your entire salvation for that matter, the great "King of the universe" always responds in kind.

2 Chronicles 30:19-20 documents this thusly: "For Hez-e-ki'-ah [king of Judah, who] had prayed for them [those at the festival of Matzoh, who had not cleansed themselves according to God's laws], 'May Adonai, who is good, pardon everyone who sets his heart on seeking God, . . . even if he hasn't undergone the purification prescribed in connection with holy things.' And the Lord hearkened to Hez-e-ki'ah, and healed the people."

My friend told me, before he hung up the phone, that he would give God a try. To the time of this writing he hadn't kept his word, and he continues his sad saga. What about you?

Yeshua on Trust in God

One of my favorite books of the Bible is Matthew. In my estimation, if you intend to drink from healing waters of the earth, it's best to go to the deepest purest source. In Matthew, blessed Yeshua described His own healing ministry in several revealing verses.

For instance, in Matthew 9:20-23, "A woman who had had a hemorrhage for twelve years approached Him from behind and touched the tzitzit on his robe. For she said to herself, 'If I can only touch his robe, I will be healed.' Yeshua turned, saw her and said, 'Courage, daughter! Your trust has healed you.' And she was instantly healed."

A few verses later Matthew 9:27-30 reads, "As Yeshua went on from there, two blind men began following him, shouting, 'Son of David! Take pity on us!' When he entered the house, the blind men came up, and Yeshua said to them, 'Do you believe that I have the power to do this?' They replied, 'Yes, sir.' Then he touched their eyes and said, 'Let it happen to you according to your trust'; and their sight was restored. . . ."

In Matthew 9:35, "Yeshua went about all the towns and villages, teaching in their synagogues, proclaiming the Good News of the Kingdom, and healing every kind of disease and weakness."

He summoned his twelve disciples in Matthew 10:1, "and gave them authority to drive out unclean spirits and to heal every kind of disease and weakness."

"These twelve Yeshua sent out with the following instructions: 'Don't go into the territory of the Gentiles, and don't enter any town in Sa-mar'i-tans, but go rather to the lost sheep of the house of Isra'el. As you go, proclaim, "The Kingdom of Heaven is near," heal the sick, raise the dead, cleanse those afflicted with leprosy, expel demons. You have received without paying, so give without asking payment. Don't take money . . . be as prudent as snakes and as harmless as doves. . . . For it will not be just you speaking, but the Spirit of your heavenly Father speaking through you.'"(Matthew 10:5-20)

Later in Matthew 15:22-28, Yeshua performed additional healings for which he credited trust in God. "A woman from Kena'an who was living there came to him, pleading. 'Sir, have pity on me. Son of David! My daughter is cruelly held under the power of demons!' But Yeshua did not say a word to her. Then his disciples came to him and urged him, 'Send her away, because she is following us and keeps pestering us with her crying.' He said, 'I was sent only to the lost sheep of the house of Isra'el.' But she came, fell at his feet and said, 'Sir, help me!' He answered, 'It is not right to take the children's food and toss it to their pet dogs.' She said, 'That is true, sir, but even the dogs eat the leftovers that fall from their master's table.' Then Yeshua answered her, 'Lady, you are a person of great trust. Let your desire be granted.' And her daughter was healed at that very moment.

"Yeshua left there and went along the shore of Lake Kinneret. He climbed a hill and sat down; and large crowds came to him, bringing with them the lame, the blind, the crippled, the mute, and many others. They laid them at his feet, and he healed them.

The people were amazed as they saw mute people speaking, crippled people cured, lame people walking, and blind people seeing; and they said prayers glorifying the God of Isra'el. . . ."

Still later in Matthew 18, Yeshua provided his famous "faith can move mountains" instruction. Prodding his students to believe in the power of God, he said "Yes! I tell you, if you have trust and don't doubt, you will not only do what was done to this fig tree; but even if you say to this mountain, 'Go and throw yourself into the sea!' it will be done."

In other words, you will receive everything you ask for in prayer, no matter what it is, "provided you have trust."

The Electromagnetic "Kingdom of Heaven"

When Yeshua told his disciples to proclaim, "The Kingdom of Heaven is near," and then in the same breath he urged them to "heal the sick, raise the dead, cleanse those afflicted with leprosy, [and] expel demons," this wasn't by accident.

Many people wish to misinterpret the phrase "The Kingdom of Heaven is near" as a temporal manifestation of God's Holy Kingdom sometime in the future, perhaps even after their death. That's not at all what Yeshua was talking about. If these temporal interpretations are so limited by time and space, then it would be impossible to perform these miracles because the Kingdom would only be "near," not *here*. That's just the point. Jesus's reference to the "Kingdom of Heaven" being near refers instead to the proximity of God's Holy Kingdom. It was so near to their touch, given their faith and trust, that they could access the healing power in it directly, and transmit it immediately into people to manifest miraculous healings.

This appraisal makes far more sense. Particularly if you think of God's Holy Kingdom as an electromagnetic state or dimension, that is so close, it virtually coexists with your own three dimensional reality. That's precisely why, through the Holy

158

Spirit—another electromagnetic matrix—you have access to everything within God's heavenly Kingdom. They obviously coexist and intermingle for the Spirit of healing to be coming from the Father, through the Son, His disciples, and people like you and me. Providing, that is, we have the *trust* required, that is, the key required to open the door to access that glorious dimension.

Furthermore, in *John G. Lake: His Life, His Sermons, His Boldness of Faith* (Kenneth Copeland Publications, Fort Worth Texas, 76192-0001), the Christian minister who the United States Government credited for having made Spokane, Washington, years ago, "the healthiest city in the world," explains how this electromagnetic healing matrix, the Judeo-Christian world calls the Holy Spirit, can be transmitted through objects such as clothing worn by anointed persons.

Minister Lake revealed, as we argued in *Healing Codes for the Biological Apocalypse*, that "Atonement through the grace of God is scientific in its application. Jesus used many methods of healing the sick. All were scientific." Today, science is pointing to electromagnetic fields, and their conductive matrices, as playing a key role in health and Spiritual communion. According to John Lake, "Science is the discovery of how God does things."

Minister Lake's book further recalled:

> Jesus laid His hands upon the sick in obedience to the law of contact and transmission. Contact of His hands with the sick . . . permitted the Spirit of God in Him to flow into the sick person.

> The sick woman who touched His clothes found that the Spirit emanated from His person. "She touched the hem of his garment [Matthew 9:20] and the Spirit flashed into her. She was made whole." This is a scientific process.

> Paul, knowing this law, laid his hands upon handkerchiefs and aprons. . . . The Spirit of God emanating from Paul transformed the handkerchiefs into storage

batteries of Holy Spirit power. When they were laid upon the sick they surcharged the body, and healing was the result. (Acts 19:12.)

This demonstrates, firstly: The Spirit of God is a tangible substance, a heavenly materiality. Secondly: It is capable of being stored in the substance of cloth as demonstrated in the garments of Jesus or the handkerchiefs of Paul. Thirdly: It will transmit power . . . His love and power in them redeems them from sin and sickness . . . and establishes the Kingdom of Heaven.

In *Healing Codes for the Biological Apocalypse,* Dr. Puleo and I relay much of the science behind this healing Spirit in those who serve God. It also reveals and discusses God's heavenly tones that need to be known, further investigated, and used here on Earth, as God uses them in heaven, to facilitate personal and world healing.

Words from the Lips

The physics of sound, including that of the spoken word, incorporates electromagnetic phenomenon including waves moving through space. That space is likewise composed of energy grids or matrices. That God created man "in his image," and used His spoken Word to give form to that image, suggests that as children of God, we humans were likewise empowered to create in a similar fashion—through the spoken word. That's precisely how prayer works to produce miracles.

In the last sections I touched upon God's covenant to make you healthy, keep you that way, as well as prosper, so long as you place Him first, and obey His laws. Then I relayed the powerful role that trust plays in all relationships, particularly in your relationship to God. As Yeshua said, "By your trust in Him are you healed." Notice each time the Prince of Peace directed a miraculous healing, He did so by first confirming the person's trust in God, and had them *articulate* through their lips their faith.

In 2 Kings 2:20-22, the prophet Elisha, "went out to the source of the polluted water, threw salt in it, and said, 'This is what Adonai says: "I have healed this water; it will no longer cause death or miscarrying."'" The water was healed and has remained healed to this day, in keeping with Elisha's *spoken word*."

A fundamental tenant underlying religious prayer is that faith, placed by the breath of prayerful words into the Holy Spirit—which is directly connected to God, has the power to create that which is faithfully and righteously desired. Underlying this miraculous phenomenon is the basic physics of sound.

I have mentioned the word "righteousness" a couple of times in the same breath as faithfulness. In relation to creating miracles through prayer, both are required. Previously, I mentioned "righteousness" was "right standing with God." Let me define righteousness a bit more using John G. Lake's words as it relates to prayer power:

> Righteousness is simply God's rightness. God's rightness in a man's soul; God's rightness in a man's spirit; God's rightness in a man's body. In order that man may be right or righteous, God imparts to man the power of His Spirit. That Spirit contains such marvelous and transforming grace that when received into the nature of man, the marvelous process of regeneration is set in motion and man becomes thereby a new creation in Christ Jesus.

> The deepest call of our nature is the one that will find the speediest answer. People pray, something happens. If they pray again, something still deeper occurs within their nature, and they find a new prayer. The desire is obtained.

Proverbs 12:18-22 and 13:17 teaches that "Idle talk can pierce like a sword, but the tongue of the wise can heal. Truthful words will stand forever . . ." This book goes on to say that "Lying lips are an abomination to God, but those who deal faithfully are His delight. . . . He who despises a word [some Bibles say 'a wicked messenger'] falls into trouble; but a faithful envoy ['who respects a command', including God's laws] is healed."

Yeshua, again in Matthew 12:36, goes one step further in asserting the association between creating your reality and the spoken word. Using a parable, the Son of man explains that God's "judgement" of you occurs instantaneously in response to your words. Here's the passage:

> If you make a tree good, its fruit will be good; and if you make a tree bad, its fruit will be bad; for a tree is known by its fruit. You snakes! How can you who are evil say anything good? For the mouth speaks what overflows from the heart. The good person brings forth good things from his store of good, and the evil person brings forth evil things from his store of evil. Moreover, I tell you this; on the Day of Judgment people will have to give account for every careless word they have spoken; for by your own words you will be acquitted, and by your own words you will be condemned.

How could the spoken word so quickly and thoroughly bear fruit and judgment? According to modern science, these phenomena are best explained considering the electromagnetics and harmonics of sound. That is, the spiritual resonance of the spoken words playing on the frequency matrix of the Holy Spirit connected to God's Heavenly Kingdom.

In *The Secret Life of Plants*, I learned that plant physiology reacts dramatically to the sound of the human voice. Words, both positive and negative, produce profound changes in water flow dynamics, and the basic physiological functions upon which plant life rests. Plants, like humans, are composed mostly of water. In Chapter 6 of this book, I described a bit of the electromagnetics and structure of clustered water. In *Healing Codes for the Biological Apocalypse*, I relayed the fact that Dr. Lee Lorenzen had impregnated his C-400 clustered water formula with the "528" frequency of "miracles" according to these newly revealed

Bible codes. Clearly, Dr. Lorenzen explains, water molecules that hold this six-sided, Divine geometric ring form, function as electromagnetic memory units capable of transmitting memories of sound, color, and light frequencies to humans and plants. This, again, is the science upon which the entire field of homeopathic medicine rests.

A good example of this is in *The Message from Water: Take a Look At Ourselves* (CellCore International, 1999). The book's author, the renowned Japanese physician, Dr. Masaru Emoto, published full color photomicrographs (i.e., 20,000 magnification pictures) of beautiful six-sided ringed crystal molecular water clusters which formed from distilled water from the sound of words of love, appreciation, or classical music. Four of these incredible pictures are reprinted (in black and white) in figures 7.1 and 7.2. Alternatively, Dr. Emoto showed that "heavy metal music," or condemning words, caused beautiful regularly-shaped water clusters to explode into shapeless messes. Dr. Emoto explained, as Yeshua had, that words and music coming from "good" or "evil" hearts can profoundly affect human health and energy. These effects are mediated by water.

Dr. Emoto concluded, "Indeed, there is nothing more important than love and gratitude in this world. Just by expressing love and gratitude, the water around us and in our bodies changes so beautifully. We want to apply this in our daily lives, don't we?"

In summary, words from your lips, like those of your Father's powerfully creative Words, are electromagnetic messages that have a profound impact on who you are, and what you will become. Virtually your entire reality, the life you live, as well as your life in the hereafter, is dramatically affected by your spoken words.

This makes sense for the Holy child of God that you are. Your Father, never forget, created you in His image through His spoken Word. That is, using His imagination much like you use

Fig. 7.1. Six-Sided Ringed Clustered Water Molecules Formed From Love versus Hate

Love/Appreciation

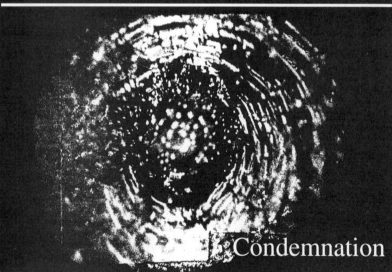

Condemnation

Photographs taken at 20,000 magnification show the results of "words of love and appreciation" versus the harsh and condemning words "You fool!" on the structural transformation of originally cube-shaped distilled water. The upper photo shows a six-sided, ringed, snowflake-like, clustered water with a hexagon at its core and a "Star of David" externally. Research shows this configuration is consistently found in healing waters studied around the world. Source: Emoto, M. *The Message from Water: Telling Us to Take a Look at Ourselves*. Irvine, CA: CellCore International, 1999)

Fig. 7.2. Flash-Frozen Water Structurally Transformed By "Clasical" versus "Heavy Metal Music"

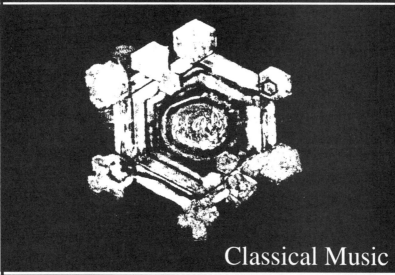

Classical Music

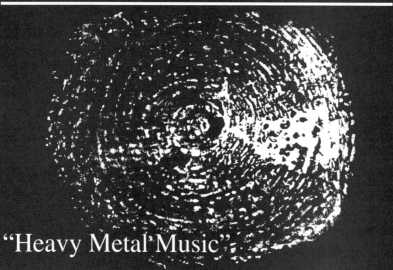

"Heavy Metal Music"

Photographs taken at 20,000 magnification show the results of "classical music" versus the harsh "heavy metal music" on the structural transformation of originally cube-shaped distilled water. The upper photo shows a six-sided, ringed, snowflake-like, clustered water typical of the healing wells studied around the world. The lower photo shows a remarkably different chaotic structure. Which would you choose for your body composed of more than eighty percent water? Source: Emoto, M. *The Message from Water: Telling Us to Take a Look at Ourselves*. Irvine, CA: CellCore International, 1999) yours to guide creativity, He and His Word simultaneously expressed the image of you into the electromagnetic matrix of the universe to create you. As a loving parent, He wanted you to be likewise empowered to co-create, from a shapeless Spiritual matrix, everything beautiful. So he gave you lips, a tongue, and the creative breath containing oxygen that delivers the energy needed to assure existence. That's why Yeshua said, "for by your own words you will be acquitted, and by your own words you will be condemned." Thus, you need to take responsibility for the awesome power and confidence God gave you to co-create peace on earth as it is in Heaven.

You can bank on this God given gift—your creative power, through prayer and your spoken word—to produce miraculous healings and other pleasantries in life. Speak supportive and loving words, and sing your prayers of hope, praise, glory, and positive vision into the Holy Spirit. Through this magnificent electromagnetic matrix of creative possibilities, from *His* Heavenly Kingdom, you will be blessed with the miracles you need to walk with Him in health and prosperity.

Chapter 8.
Miraculous Healings, Faith, Forgiveness, and Love

"Commit your way to Adonai;
trust in him, and he will act.
He will make your vindication shine forth like light,
the justice of your cause like the noonday sun."

Psalms 37:5-6
The Complete Jewish Bible

There is no doubt in my mind that the same auditory electromagnetic mechanism used by God to create the universe,
and available to you to co-create with Him, will produce the
Great Healing—the Messianic Age of peace, love, and enlight-
enment. As explained in *Healing Codes for the Biological
Apocalypse*, the 144,000 humble, scholarly, and empowered servants of God, first prophesied in the Bible, are currently being
assembled. They will sing the specific notes, at least six of which
God has already revealed, just the right frequencies of sound,
that will miraculously and instantaneously revert this planet and
its people back to God's Holy Domain. It is, therefore, a great
time for celebrating. This title, *Healing Celebrations* was derived
in this Spirit of prophecy and expectation. The power of God is
coming on so strong, even at the time of this writing, that it will
be impossible for anyone, even the evil Adversary, to resist its
sweet sound and Spirited effects. The Holy Spirit of peace will
come on so powerfully that those in dissonance will implode immediately from their own discord. Those in Divine Harmony will

be forever uplifted in the Rauch HaKodesh, the Holy Spirit, of everlasting peace, love, and light.

There is a passage in 2 Chronicles 5:11-14 that paints a very similar picture. After King Solomon had finished building his father David's great tribute to God—the Temple—that the Lord gratefully inhabited, it was time for celebrating. Here's what occurred as translated from the original Hebrew in the *Complete Jewish Bible*:

> When the cohanim came out of the Holy Place (for all the cohanim who were present had consecrated themselves; they didn't keep to their divisions; also the L'vi'im who were the singers, all of them — Asaf, Heman, Y'dutun and their sons and relatives — dressed in fine linen, with cymbals, lutes and lyres, stood on the east side of the alter; and with them 120 cohanim sounding trumpets), then, when the trumpeters and singers were playing in concord, to be heard harmoniously praising and thanking Adonai, and they lifted their voices together with the trumpets, cymbals, and other musical instruments to praise Adonai: "for he is good, for his grace continues forever" — then, the house, the house of Adonai, was filled with a cloud; so that because of the cloud, the cohanim could not stand up to perform their service; for the glory of Adonai filled the house of God.

In other words, the rabbis and entire congregation were blown off their feet by the surging presence of God called to the scene by prayer, songs, and notes of praise. That's all it will take to miraculously and instantaneously deliver this planet, and its people, from the grips of evil to the sustenance of God.

Indeed, it's time for celebrating. By following the recommendations provided in this book, you will build your "temple of God," your body, to be inhabited by Him, His Son, and the Holy Spirit. The power of this trinity within you will uplift you so immeasurably into the Kingdom of Heaven, that like the rabbis described above, you will be completely overwhelmed and knocked over by this Spirit of Renewal.

Faith and Provisions

By now, it should be apparent that the first provision you need to make for this celebratory period is to develop your faith in God. This is the first provision necessary to experience miraculous healings and be blessed beyond measure. This is intimated in Exodus 33:12-15 wherein Moses bade the Lord to keep by His people's side as they prepared and then embarked on their journey to the promised land. In fact, throughout Exodus, God's chosen people were encouraged to make preparations for their upcoming spiritual and physical journeys.

Later, in Numbers 11:17, God became really perturbed by the Hebrews reticence towards following His laws. So he instructed Moses to, "Tell the people: 'Consecrate yourselves in preparation for tomorrow' . . . "

The word consecrate is very important. Defined in *Webster's Dictionary*, it means a "sacred" act "to induct a person into a permanent office with a religious rite . . . to devote irrevocably to the worship of God by a solemn ceremony. . . ." In other words, God told His people that the act of preparing for any coming event is a sacred Holy process. When you make preparations to receive or achieve anything, the glory must *first* be given to God because of the Holy nature of His manifesting process. Remember from Deuteronomy 8:17, it is God who grants you the power to get everything, including wealth, according to His covenant, "which He swore to your ancestors, as is happening even today." So, if you want to claim your part of His Kingdom, solemnly swear to make Him Lord over your life.

Yeshua, too, spoke often of making provisions for the Kingdom of Heaven to be here on earth, manifesting His glory and abundance for all his disciples. A great prescription is found in Luke 11:9-10. Here Yeshua encourages you to "keep asking, and it will be given to you; keep seeking, and you will find; keep knocking, and the door will be opened to you. For everyone who goes on asking receives; and he who goes on seeking finds; and to him who continues knocking, the door will be opened."

Likewise in 2 Chronicles 20:20, King Y'hoshafat of Judah told the people of Jerusalem to prepare themselves to succeed with faith in God. He said, "Have faith [trust or believe] in Adonai your God, and you will be safe [or upheld]. Have faith in His prophets, and you will succeed."

Making provisions, first spiritual, and then physical, for anything new, including dramatic healings, is one of the most important steps you can take to claim your Heavenly treasures. Healing and wellness comes out of your wholeness and association with God who is complete in every way—lacking nothing—and in total balance. By simply preparing yourself to be likewise, and blessed by His grace through your faith in Him, your actions create the movement and continued motivation in the direction to manifest the wholeness and wellness you seek.

According to James 2:22; 2:26, your actions taken in effort to manifest a healthier and more prosperous life through faith, actually *complete* the faith. "Indeed," James wrote, "just as the body without a spirit is dead, so too faith without action is dead."

In other words, for the doors to open, you need to step up to the door and knock or kick it in. Sometimes that means putting on a pair of running shoes, or army boots, or taking a battering ram to the front gate. In every situation, if you walk with God, you'll get the guidance you need to select the correct provisions you need, and course of action to take.

Provision by Tithing

Parenthetically, a provision for prosperity is God's Holy tithe. Lots of people suffer physically due to monetary deprivation. Like healing, it is not God that deprives you from wealth. It is you, and your lack of trust and righteousness in following His commands.

Regarding supernaturally created prosperity, the Lord ordered His people in Leviticus 27:30 to set aside one tenth of their first fruits in respect to His glory and sustenance. "A tithe of everything from the land, whether grain from the soil or fruit from the trees, belongs to the Lord, it is holy to God."

In Deuteronomy 26:12-14, God tells you what to do with the tithe—His ten percent of your income. "When you have finished setting aside a tenth of all your produce . . . you shall give it to the Levite, the alien, the fatherless and the widow, so that they may eat in your towns and be satisfied." Then, once you have prayed to God to determine which of the above sanctified recipients are to receive His money (or other valued earnings), "say to the Lord your God: 'I have removed from my house the sacred portion and have given it to the Levite, the alien, the fatherless and the widow, according to all you commanded. I have not turned aside from your commands nor have I forgotten any of them. I have not eaten any of the sacred portion while I was in mourning, nor have I removed any of it while I was unclean, nor have I offered any of it to the dead. I have obeyed the Lord my God; I have done everything you commanded me. [Therefore,] look down from heaven, your holy dwelling place, and bless your people Israel and the land you have given us as you promised on oath to our forefathers, . . . [a] land flowing with milk and honey.'"

As the above reference notes, and as I have stated repeatedly in this book, God is obliged by His contract with your forefathers, beginning with Abraham, to prosper and heal you if you do what He requests, *including this tithe.* Your land will flow "with milk and honey" if you do. "See if I won't open for you the floodgates of heaven and pour out for you a blessing far beyond your needs. For your sakes I will forbid the devourer to destroy the yield from your soil; and your vine will not lose its fruit before harvest-time," said God. "All nations will call you happy, for you will be a land of delights." All with respect to the tithe.

As a personal testimony to the power in following this lesser known law, my wife, Jackie, and I had not been tithers. We simply rationalized our many social contributions as sufficient for warranting admission into the "Kingdom of Heaven" wherein prosperity is commonplace. Recently, however, following months of unsuccessful efforts to get our business's credit card debt down to zero from $30,000, our hopes seemed dismal. I had gone from September through mid December, typically my greatest earning period, without making a dent in our balance. Then a friend explained to us the Spiritual dynamic of tithing. "A tithe into the Gospel returns a hundred fold," she said (based on Matthew 19:29 and Mark 10:30).

"But everything we do is a contribution to God and humanity!" Jackie replied. "We put all of our money into projects that help people wake up and be saved, not only from man-made risks, but saved Spiritually as well."

"That's not the way God's law reads," our friend returned. "You have got to take *ten percent of your first fruits*. That's God's money! Pray on where it should go. Then send it there. Then you can come before the Lord in prayer and ask him to handle your credit card debt."

So we did just that. We calculated our gross income over the previous three months, and multiplied by ten percent. Then we prayed for guidance and were Divinely inspired to write checks to various people and ministries.

THE VERY NEXT DAY, a miracle happened. Panicked by our diluted checking account, Jackie decided to begin reconciling her end-of-the-year bank records. Lo and behold, she realized, she had made an unprecidented $32,000 mistake in our favor! She immediately wrote the checks to pay off our credit card debts.

One day later, on the Sunday before Christmas, we attended a new church by invitation of a gracious neighbor. The chapel was packed with more than 800 people assembled to hear a special holiday concert. An usher escorted our family to an open pew section, and we sat down. Moments later the pastor said, "Welcome! This is, indeed, a special holiday season. It's a time for giving. Please look down at your Bible rack and pick up the red card in front of you." So I looked down and picked up the red card.

"Now, please raise your hand if you have a red card," he said. So I raised my hand. Oddly, there were only two other people in the entire assembly whose hands were raised.

"We want to give you folks a special prize, a gift from our church, in the spirit of Christmas."

That blew me away. You see, prior to that moment, I had never won anything in my life! I used to pride myself in telling people, "Oh, I never win anything. God always blesses me in other ways." Suddenly I realized that winning something *is* a Godly blessing that I open myself to receiving when I follow His laws *entirely*. The fact is, more abundant prosperity, like health, manifests supernaturally from God, the source of everything, the wider you open the "flood gate of Heaven."

Thus, I now understand and share God's ways, and His joy, in giving. As Yeshua's emissary, John, wrote to his friend Gaius (3 John 2): "Dear friend, I am praying that everything prosper with you and that you be in good health [as you are] faithful . . . to the truth. Nothing gives me greater joy than hearing that my children are living in the truth."

Forgiveness of Sin

As the word implies, everything in God's Heavenly Kingdom is for giving. Even eternal grace for those who, in ignorance of His laws and ways, allow themselves to be deceived. God forgives even those who sin against Him and His people. He ultimately gave His precious Son to be sacrificed for the cause of human freedom from Babylonian tyranny. Everything that comes naturally to the earth, God gave freely for use and enjoyment by His people. From the air you breathe, and the water you drink, to the heat and sun that makes your plants grow. All of this God continues to bestow on you and humanity, despite the best efforts of evil ones to harness, regulate, pollute, and/or destroy His great gifts.

It is humanly hard to integrate absolute forgiveness as a way of life. Interesting that by the time you do, you barely need to apply it. What do I mean? Consider the following:

You have certainly found it difficult to forgive certain people in your life for having harmed you in one or more ways you consider "unforgivable." Nearly everyone holds some grudge against someone else.

It is usually only after you have matured, overcome the injury, or transmuted/transcended the emotional pain that you are able to forgive and move ahead in your life. In retrospect, your lack of forgiveness actually hurts you more than the one who harmed you. Likewise, when you harbor anger against another person, you actually *lose yourself to that anger.* In essence, you are more that person than yourself at the time you are ruminating about how bad that person is, and how much they harmed you. Their badness fills your mind and evicts all goodness of spirit that you could have experienced at that moment. What a waste of time and energy! No wonder God wants you to learn forgiveness as a way of life.

Forgiveness, in fact, demonstrates Divine love and unity because, now get this, the only reason someone could have harmed you to begin with, given God's covenant of prosperity and protection, is if you had not walked with Him in Righteousness, in truth, and in His Kingdom of Divine protection, in the first place. Did you get it? (Read the sentence again until it sinks in.)

Couple this lesson with the law of Divine judgement—"as you sow, so shall you reap"—and you can better understand why God desires you to forgive sins against you, as He forgives the sins against Him. Through your forgiveness, you too are forgiven. You are, in all practical terms, forgiving yourself when you forgive others, and reinventing/recreating yourself as a Divinely inspired being.

Thus, what kind of world could be made if everyone consistently practiced forgiveness? If everyone always forgave others, relying instead on God's fairness and His laws for settling disputes (See Matthew 5:21-7:27.), then everyone connected with these issues would be forgiven *and* all would be elevated a notch toward Divine unity and Righteousness. Did you get that? If not, let this be your homework. Read this section again until you integrate it.

This understanding of forgiveness explains why blessed Yeshua said in Matthew 5:39-48, "Do not resist an evil person. If someone strikes you on the cheek, turn to him the other also. And if someone wants to sue you and take your tunic, let him have your cloak as well." His advice comes from the knowledge that we are all in this together, "on earth as it is in Heaven."

"You have heard that our fathers were told, 'Love your neighbor . . . and hate your enemy,'" Yeshua continued. "But I tell you, love your enemies! Pray for those who persecute you! Then you will become children of your Father in heaven. For he makes his sun shine on good and bad people alike, and he sends rain to the righteous and the unrighteous alike. What reward do you get if you love only those who love you? Why, even tax-collectors do that! And if you are friendly only to your friends, are you doing anything out of the ordinary? Even the Gentiles do that! Therefore, be perfect, just as your Father in heaven is perfect!"

Clearly, that is perfection, to which we should all aspire, work, and pray to achieve.

Indeed, forgiveness of sin, yours and other people's, is such an important part of this perfection—God's plan for planetary salvation—that John the Baptist's mute father Zacharias, the king of Judea, filled with the Holy Spirit, suddenly spoke prophesying the coming of Yeshua for this specific purpose. His son John, as had previously been prophesied (Malachi 3:1, Isaiah 40:3), would "go before the Lord to prepare his way by spreading the knowledge among his people that *deliverance comes by having sins forgiven through our God's most tender mercy*, which causes the Sunrise to visit us from Heaven, to shine upon those in darkness, living in the shadow of death, and to guide our feet into the paths of peace." (Luke 1:76-79)

In fact, the very rational plan that God realized must be actualized, was to provide a Royal Sacrifice in order to make eternal forgiveness and salvation available to *all* people. God had close to struck out, time after time, trying to keep His chosen people on track following His laws. The old testament records this and His frustrations with His first covenant. He realized that even His chosen people were often not willing to make all the sacrifices called for in Moses's Levitical Laws (as relayed in Leviticus, Numbers, and Deuteronomy). Many, if not most, of these sacrifices to atone for sin became practically impossible with time. Today, they would be virtually impossible to accomplish given the frequent animal sacrifices and blood rituals required under God's old covenant. Therefore, it makes most exquisite sense that God needed a supreme sacrifice to substitute for His old impractical and largely neglected covenant. A sacrifice so great that its power would endure throughout eternity and cover people, like a spiritual insurance policy, against their violations of truth, justice, faith, and love.

This is much like the message that Sha'ul, Apostle Paul, relayed. On the road to Damascus, the strictly religious Pharisee, acting with the "full authority and power of the high priest," intending to persecute Yeshua, suddenly "saw a light from heaven, brighter than the sun, shining around" him and his traveling companions. (See Acts 26:12-17.) It was Yeshua who came to "deliver" him from his deceivers and Babylonian deception.

"I am sending you to open their eyes," said the Messiah, "so that they will turn from darkness into light, from the power of the Adversary to God, and thus receive *forgiveness* of sins and a place among those who have been separated for holiness by putting their trust in me."

Social Unity Through Forgiveness

Paul continued clarifying Yeshua's instructions, including this power of forgiveness. Obviously disappointing the Pharisees—the most religious Hebrew rabbis included—Paul attempted to relieve their "pain." In his letter to them in 2 Corinthians, Paul beautifully relays the same truth of relationship between social unity, God, and forgiveness of sin. In bidding the rabbis farewell, Paul wrote:

> So I made up my mind that I would not pay you another painful visit. For if I cause you pain, who is left to make me happy except the people I have pained? Indeed, this is why I wrote as I did — so that when I came, I would not have to be pained by those who ought to be making me happy; for I had enough confidence in all of you to believe that unless I could be happy, none of you could be happy either. I wrote to you with a greatly distressed and anguished heart, and with many tears, not in order to cause you pain, but to get you to realize how very much I love you.
>
> Now if someone has been a cause of pain, it is not I whom he has pained, but, in some measure — I don't want to overstate it — all of you. For such a person the punishment already imposed on him by the majority is sufficient, so that now you should do the opposite — forgive him, encourage him, comfort him. Otherwise such a person might be swallowed up in overwhelming depression. So I urge you to show that you really do love him. The reason I wrote you was to see if you would pass the test, to see if you would fully obey me.

> Anyone you forgive, I forgive too. For indeed, whatever
> I have forgiven, if there has been anything to forgive,
> has been for your sake in the presence of the Messiah
> so that we will not be taken advantage of by the Adver-
> sary — for we are quite aware of his schemes!

During the first *Healing Celebrations* event that Dr. Valerie Saxion and I hosted in Portland, Oregon at the start of the new millennium, a young man with AIDS came to us for prayer and healing. He explained that his father had sexually abused him when he was a child, and hating his dad for that, he had never forgiven him. As he stood before us that day, he relayed that two years earlier he had wished death upon his father. Within six months, he testified, his father died of cancer. Feeling desperately guilty for his lack of forgiveness, and feeling that he was unforgivable, the young man told us that he was moved to contract AIDS because he felt that his life was not worth living. Minutes later, after prayer, having forgiven his father for his abuses, and having forgiven himself for his sins against his dad, himself, and God, the man's countenance and posture dramatically changed. He was greatly healed by the Spirit of forgiveness and the eternal salvation that those precious moments brought.

A Miracle of Faith

Jo, a spirited woman in her thirties also came to our first *Healing Celebrations* event needing a miracle. A thyroid tumor, the size of an orange, protruded from the left side of her neck. The goiter, her doctors said, caused her thyroxin levels to go "sky high." The hormone was responsible for her near cardiac arrest condition. Her heart rate had escalated to a frenzied 138 beats-per-minute. This risk, her doctors said, made an operation impossible. Her only "medical option" was to undergo radiation. If successful, chemotherapy would be needed for the rest of her life. Even then, she was expected to die prematurely.

Having more faith in God than her doctors, Jo placed her trust and life in God's hands. She refused to take the drugs her doctors ordered, hopped into her car, and drove from central Wyoming to Portland, Oregon to attend our *Healing Celebrations* program. Here, she fully expected God to deliver a merciful miracle.

When we called people to the front of the room for prayer and healing, Jo was among the first on her feet. She raced to the front of the line, and soon stood between Dr. Saxion and myself. A team of prayer warriors lent their support as Valerie placed her hands on Jo's face. I braced her lower spine with my right hand in case she fell out in the Spirit. My left hand went to the back of Jo's neck.

Everyone prayed intensely for a few minutes as God's Holy Spirit fell upon us. The healing force became so intense that Jo suddenly began to speak in tongues—something she had never done before.

Then Valerie's hands fell naturally onto Jo's neck. Her left hand gently caressed Jo's goiter. At that moment, my left hand became hot. I felt the sweat beading from my palm onto the back of Jo's neck. Valerie's loving hands began to vibrate. "They became *burning* hot," she later recalled, just as Jo began to feel something happening inside.

An instant later, in a futile effort to remain calm, Jo shouted, "It's disappearing." Valerie instantly felt the large mass dissolve in her hand. Within seconds the goiter completely disappeared.

Overcome with joy, to the amazement of more than a hundred witnesses, Jo exclaimed, "It's gone! It's gone! It's totally gone! I'm healed!!!" She screamed euphorically, and danced around for several minutes crying and hugging people in ecstatic celebration.

"I walked in that anointing for ten hours," she later told us. "I just knew I was going to be healed. My husband still can't believe it. Today my pulse is down to 69 and the goiter is completely gone."

"Daughter, your faith has healed you," Yeshua said (Luke 8:48). "Go in peace."

A Final Note on Trust

Paul summarized the basic truth regarding the awesome loving power of God and the sacrifice He and Yeshua made for personal and world healing. In Ephesians 7-15 he wrote, "In union with him, through the shedding of his blood, we are set free — our sins are forgiven; . . . [I]n union with him we were given an inheritance . . . Furthermore, you who heard the message of truth, the Good News offering you deliverance, and put your *trust* in the Messiah were *sealed* by him with the promised Rauch Ha-Kodesh [Holy Spirit], who guarantees our inheritance until we come into possession of it and thus bring him praise commensurate with his glory. . . ."

"I pray that from the treasures of his glory he will empower you with inner strength by his Spirit, so that the Messiah may live in your hearts through your trusting. Also I pray that you will be rooted and founded in love, so that you, with all God's people, will be given strength to grasp the breadth, length, and depth of the Messiah's love, yes, to know it, even though it is beyond all knowing, so that you will be filled with all the fullness of God.

"Now to him who by his power working in us is able to do far beyond anything we ask or imagine, to him be glory in the Messianic Community and in the Messiah Yeshua from generation to generation forever. *Amen*." (Ephesians 3:16-21)

A Final Note on Love

Daily I receive dozens of letters from well-wishers who attach special articles, books, tapes, and other documents for my perusal. One came just in time for this book's final section. Paul James and his lovely wife, Waleen—author of the book *The Myth of Immunization*, sent us a book compiled by a study group associated with the Edgar Cayce Foundation. A large section of *A Search for God* dealt with "The Power of Love." It beautifully summarized much of this book's wisdom. Here's what they wrote:

> Love is the force that uplifts and inspires mankind. Children starve without it. Men and women wither and decay when it is lacking. It costs nothing, yet its value cannot be measured by material standards. It can lift a wretched human being from the miry clay of despair and set his feet upon the solid rock of respectability and service.

> Love is that inexplicable force which brought Jesus to earth so that through Him the way back to the Father might be made plain to the children of men. It caused the Father to give His Son that whosoever believes might have eternal life. Love is that dynamic force which brings into manifestation all things. It is the healing force, the cleansing force, and the force that blesses all things we touch. With our hearts filled with love we will see only goodness and purity in everybody and in everything. In the beginning love looked upon the earth and saw that it was good and blessed it.

> As love is God, it is, therefore, our abundant supply. Do we lack? Do we love? Do we allow conditions to keep us from the realization of the presence of God? If so, how can we expect the flow of abundance, when we are keeping the channel blocked by our thoughts and attitudes? We are standing in the way of our own success.

> When conditions arise which seem hard to endure, if we would realize that we are workers together with God and that each condition is perhaps some problem in our lives that must be met and overcome, we might stop and count our blessings instead of counting our hardships. Only with our hearts filled with love—love for conditions, love for people, love for God—can we fully realize this.

> Life is growth. We never can grow in knowledge and understanding and really be channels of blessings until we have endured and conquered in ourselves just the things that we would help others to overcome. Love allows no place for

that and recognizes no evil, but sees all things working together for good. The power of love is unlimited. We alone may set the metes and bounds. We may use it constructively or selfishly. We may uplift our fellow man or crush ideals, instigate revolts, and wreck civilization. It all depends upon whether we are in love with ourselves or are willing to lay down our lives for others.

"The Father's love," the authors concluded, "is the golden thread that is woven throughout the Scriptures." His love enlarges and spreads until His whole law is fulfilled, and we are elevated by it into His Heavenly Kingdom.

In 1 Corinthians 13, Paul wrote:

I may have the gift of prophecy, I may fathom all mysteries, know all things, have all faith—enough to move mountains; but if I lack Love, I am nothing. . . .

Love is patient and kind, not jealous, not boastful, not proud, rude or selfish, not easily angered, and it keeps no record of wrongs. Love does not gloat over other people's sins but takes its delight in the truth. Love always bears up, always trusts, always hopes, always endures . . . Love never ends . . . Pursue love!

Thus, the way to the Father, for continuous *Healing Celebrations*, is through love. God gave you—His Holy child—the opportunity to join Him in oneness, wholeness, and health. His way was heralded by Yeshua for "those who have eyes to see and ears to hear." Place your faith in Him, and act according to His laws and love. Then, rather than illness you will manifest health. Your trust will dispel fear and anger, and instead of taking credit yourself for the miracles you manifest, you will say "Rather, it is the Father, living in me, who is doing his work." (John 14:10)

"Then I saw another sign in heaven,
a great and wonderful one —
seven angels with the seven plagues
that are the final ones;
because with them, God's fury is finished. . . .
Those defeating the beast, its image and the number
of its name were standing by the sea of glass,
holding harps which God had given them.
They were singing the song of Moses, the servant of God,
and the song of the Lamb:

'Great and wonderful are the things you have done,
Adonai, God of heaven's armies!
Just and true are your ways,
king of the nations!
Adonai, who will not fear and glorify your name?
because you alone are holy.
All nations will come and worship before you,
for your righteous deeds have been revealed.'"

Revelation 15:1-4,
The Complete Jewish Bible

Healing Celebrations

Appendix

In several earlier chapters, references were made to risks associated with vaccinations for children and adults. Many people
believe that vaccinations are safe and "mandatory" for school
and/or workplace attendance. They are clearly deceived in most
cases. Vaccines are not "mandatory" in most American states that
allow for personal, religious, and/or medical exemptions. Furthermore, the practice of vaccination is far from safe. In fact, if
you were to seriously consider the suppressed facts you would
likely conclude that the alleged benefits of vaccination do not
outweigh the severe, extensive, and common risks.

For parents who elect to forego these risks, respecting God
and His blessings, among which are health and natural immunity, the following pages include Bible verses that should be cop-
ied and then attached to your vaccination waiver or declination
form(s).

Vaccination: The UnGodly Practice

The following Bible excerpts serve as a supplement to the
ninety-minute audiotape entitled, *Horowitz "On Vaccines."* This
tape provides a lengthy discussion on a citizen's right to refuse
vaccination for spiritual and religious reasons, and ways to avoid
vaccinations and assertively respond to coercive vaccine propo-
nents and shot administrators. Moreover, the tape presents stunning admissions by vaccine industry experts, including 1998
Sabin Gold Medal of Honor awardee Dr. Maurice Hilleman, and
others who admit to the contaminated and deadly nature of many
of our most trusted vaccines.

Biblical support for those who wish to avoid vaccinations for spiritual and religious reasons includes the following law prohibiting genetic engineering or the use of its products:

> **Leviticus 19:19** Ye shall keep my statutes. Thou shalt not let thy cattle gender with a diverse kind: thou shalt not sow thy field with mingled seed: neither shall a garment mingled of linen [plant] and woolen [animal] come upon thee.

Relevant reasons for God's warning in this regard include the fact that bovine (cow) fetal serum is commonly used in the manufacturing process of vaccines. So are monkey kidney cells, chicken embryo parts, bacterial or viral genetic materials—RNA and DNA, as well as yeast and human proteins. Using the example of cows, bovine fetal serum is mixed with bacteria or viral particles and other vaccine ingredients including toxic metals such as mercury, aluminum, and immune destructive chemicals. Thus, proteins and genetic materials from the cattle, viruses, and bacteria are mixed before these particles are injected into you or your children. Once the vaccine ingredients, including foreign RNA and DNA, and genetically engineered bacteria and/or viruses, or their parts, enter your blood, they may cause genetic mutations of *your* cells. Then you have sown thy bloodstream "with mingled seed" that not only taxes your immune system further, but may cause the development of cancer cells as well. These may go on to become full blown cancers, particularly in the presence of a weakened immune system made weak by vaccine "adjuvents."

Likewise, this cross species transfer of infectious particles often initiates autoimmune diseases, as discussed in Chapter 4 of this book. These are major reasons why vaccination is an "unGodly practice."

Your blood contains vital white blood cell body guards (i.e., lymphocytes) that provide for surveillance and destructive responses against cancer cells and malignant tumors. Therefore, over taxing these cells, as vaccinations often do, is unclean and unhealthy. Elsewhere in the Bible, God recommends that you maintain your blood clean and healthy.

Integrating this knowledge further, some vaccines are made from "pooling" human blood taken from people, including social drop-outs and drug addicts, who were exposed to various infectious agents (e.g., bacteria and viruses). Once vaccine makers have these people's blood, their laboratory technicians separate their serum from the whole cells, and then this serum is mixed and used to make the final vaccines.

This was the case with the hepatitis B vaccine that was given to gay men in New York City and Blacks in Central Africa in 1974. This vaccine, according to all the suppressed scientific evidence, as well as testimonies from insiders, most likely, initiated the international AIDS pandemic.

In essence, the routine vaccine manufacturing practice of sacrificing animals to grow infectious viruses is obviously risky. This was the case for the cancer and AIDS linked polio and hepatitis B vaccines. Merck vaccine makers took dead or dying animals' tissues, including their blood, in an effort to extract these infectious agents. Then they mixed these animal incubated contaminants with human blood. This blood ultimately got mixed to make the final vaccine. In this manner, cross-species transmission of infectious agents most easily and commonly occurred. This practice continues today. According to the Bible, this is a sin.

There are several Bible references to the importance of maintaining clean blood. A few of these are listed below along with other relevant verses:

Lamentations 4:13-15 foreshadows the AIDS pandemic, and other current and coming plagues. It also relays the fear and avoidance surrounding HIV-positive and other infected, sick, and dying people. As you read the first paragraph, consider the fact that religious leaders are encouraging their followers to get vaccinated. Many are even inviting "public health" nurses and vaccine administrators into their congregations to deliver the toxic, and too often lethal, doses:

> It happened because of the sins of her prophets and the offenses of her priests (and rabbis),who, within her walls, shed the blood of the righteous.
>
> They wander in the streets like the blind; they are so polluted with blood that nobody is able even to touch their clothing.
>
> Keep away! Unclean!" people shout at them, "Keep away! Away, don't touch us!" They flee, to wander here and there; but no nation allows them to stay.

Ezekial 3:18-20 provides a pretty good argument why it's important to relay these facts concerning vaccines, blood transfusions, sin, and death:

> When I say to a wicked man, 'You will surely die,' and you do not warn him or speak out to dissuade him from his evil ways in order to save his life, that wicked man will die for his sin, and I will hold you accountable for his blood.
>
> But if you do warn the wicked man and he does not turn from his wickedness or from his evil ways, he will die for his sin; but you will be saved yourself.

Ezekial 5:17 provides another blood-related warning and prophecy that may relate to recent outbreaks, particularly the hemorrhagic fever virus, Ebola. As documented in *Emerging Viruses: AIDS & Ebola—Nature, Accident or Intentional?*, this virus was apparently produced by Litton Bionetics—America's sixth leading biological weapons contracting laboratory:

> Yes, I will send famine and savage beasts upon you to leave you without children; plague and bloodshed will sweep through you; and I will bring the sword upon you. I, God, have spoken it.

Luke 13:1-5 states that those who mix human blood with the blood of sacrificed animals are "sinners." This is precisely what pharmaceutical industrialists do during the manufacture of many vaccines.

> There were present at that season some that told him of the Gallaeans, whose blood Pilate had mingled with their sacrifices.

> And Jesus answering said unto them. Suppose ye that these Galilaeans were sinners above all the Galilaeans, because they suffered such things?

Finally, Revelation provides an "End Times" prophecy in which the Kings, merchants, and wealthiest men of all the nations were deceived by "magic spells" or "sorcery." Biblical references to the practice of "magic spells" or "sorcery" comes from the Greek root word of "sorcery," that is, pharmacopeia meaning pharmacy. This "sorcery," is not only associated in the Bible with spilled and impure blood, but with the great plagues, and onslought of deadly "beasts."

Strong's Concordance Root word for "beasts" is the "Hebrew word #2416—chay—alive, raw flesh . . . appetite; in the Greek Lexicon, the Greek word #2342 for "beasts" is "therion"—"a little beast, little animal." Thus, the earth's greatest depopulation event is predicted to be associated with little beasts and the great plagues. Could these "little beasts" be bacteria, viruses, and pieces thereof—infectious microorganisms most insidiously spread throughout the world, most precisely and extensively, in contaminated blood and vaccines? That's exactly what many experts say is occurring today.

Those who "fornicated" with the devil, and stole "the blood of prophets and of God's people," would surely be severly judged by God in the last days. (See Revelation 18:23-19:2.) The Bible predicts that around the time "Babylon the great" falls, its deadly wine, also symbolic of blood, will flow out full of impurities into the "rivers and streams" that the Bible says are the earth's "people." They will likely then be infected with agents— little "beasts"—associated with great plagues that will wipe out more than a third of the world's population.

Indeed, a reasonable interpretation of these sections of Revelation include the suggestion that vaccine/pharmaceutical/blood industrialists, all largely directed by the Rockefeller family and their friends, have deceived international leaders, merchants, and the wealthy.

Finally, in Revelation, God's judgement and great wrath comes upon those who have worshiped these Babylonian idols above the Lord. Today, as modern medical science is idolized, and continues to dramatically alter the gene pools of plants, animals, microorganisms, and humans, Babylonian scientists are destroying the perfection that God created over all the earth.

Additional Bible verses of interest on these topics include:

Ezekial 14:19: Or if I [Lord God] send a pestilence into that land, and pour out my fury upon it in blood, to cut off from it man and beast.

Ezekial 16:6: And when I passed by thee, and saw thee polluted in thine own blood, I said unto thee when thou wast in thy blood, Live; yea, I said unto thee when thou wast in thy blood, Live.

Revelation 14:19-20 And the angel thrust in his sickle into the earth, and gathered the vine of the earth, and cast it into the great winepress of the wrath of God. . . . and blood flowed from the winepress.

Revelation 18:4 And I heard another voice from heaven, saying, Come out of her, my people, that ye be not partakers of her sins, and that ye receive not of her plagues.

Revelation 19:1-2 . . . the Lord our God . . . hath judged the great whore, which did corrupt the earth . . . and hath avenged the blood of his servants at her hand.

The End.

For more information regarding any of the books, tapes or products mentioned above, please contact:

Tetrahedron Publishing Group
P. O. Box 2033
Sandpoint, ID 83864
1-800-336-9266
FAX: 208-265-2775
e-mail: tetra@tetrahedron.org
or visit our website catalog at:
http://www.tetrahedron.org

The above website contains many free downloadable files concerning vaccines, cancer, autoimmune diseases, and the coming plagues.

These free articles are accessible through the "Research, News and Views" page of Tetrahedron's website. Simply click on the "FTP Public Access Files" button to review these documents.

Healing Celebrations

192

Acknowledgments

I am extremely grateful to Valerie and Jim Saxion for their friendship, spiritual guidance, and biblical scholarship over the year leading up to the writing of this book. They have been a tremendous blessing to me, my family, and everyone at Tetrahedron Publishing Group.

I also greatly appreciate the spiritual blessings provided to me by Rabbi Ralph Messer of the Messianic Community in Denver, Colorado; Minister Cal Pierce, Director of the Healing Rooms—following in the great healing traditions of John G. Lake in Spokane, Washington; The Healing Rooms staff, especially co-directors Pat and Patty for their celebratory manners, clearly relaying God's love through the Holy Spirit; and Kenneth and Gloria Copeland for their charismatic work in spreading the Gospel, and clarifying for me many grey areas in Bible interpretation.

Many thanks also go to the following people who, over the years, helped me mature spiritually. First my parents, Lily and Sieg Horowitz; my dad's father, Moses; my good friend Sherry Lane; Pamela Whitney, who first introduced me to loving Yeshua; Jackie, my wife for almost twenty years who continues to nurture and challenge me to grow spiritually; and my beautiful children Alena, Aria, and Aaron.

Thanks also go to Jim Karnstedt, James South, Lynn Kenny, Dan Kunkle, Dr. Lee Lorenzen, and Ingri Cassel for their technical knowledge and support.

Finally, I obviously want to thank and praise God for taking a mongrel like me from the Davidian and Mosaic bloodlines, living in the getto of Camden, New Jersey, and gently guiding me through the tempering processes of my life so that I might fulfill my calling to contribute something meaningful to world healing, the Messianic Age, and to celebrating in His Heavenly Kingdom.

Index

A

Absorption (of nutrients), 24
Acid forming, 49
Acid lifestyle risks, 47; foods, 50
Adam and Eve, 147
AIDS, 95; virus, 91
Alkaline, 21; minerals, 40; water, 45, 48
Alkalinizing your body, 26, 37, 38, 44, 45, 49, 50, 51. *See also*
  Deacidification
Aloe vera, 101
American Medical Association, 133
American Red Cross, 91
Amino acids, 72
Anaerobic opportunistic infections, 86
Anthrax antibody, 64
Anti-aging, 70
Antibiotic overuse, 24
Antibody production, 70; enhanced, 70
Antioxidant enzymes, 68
Apostle Paul, 128, 180. *See also* Paul and Sha'ul
Apple cider vinegar, 45
Ascorbyl-free radical, 69
Astragalis extract, 71
Autoimmune disease, 55, 59, 64
Awareness training, 20

B

B-lymphocytes, 63
Baby formulas, 80
Babylonian, 126, 174, 193; english, 126, 174, 193; scientists, 189; tyranny,
  174
Bacteria, 4, 22, 24, 25, 38, 50, 60, 61, 64, 82, 83, 87, 94, 95, 98, 104, 131,
  132, 186, 187, 192
Balch, James, 35
Beasts (associated with plagues), 94
Beta carotene, 61, 73
Bible, 1-4, 20, 20, 21, 28, 37, 38, 53, 56, 84, 85, 93-97, 105, 108, 120, 121,

J

Jenny, Hans, 116, 118
Jesus, 3, 20, 107, 151, 155, 160, 164, 180, 191, 197. *See also* Yeshua
John G. Lake: His Life, His Sermons, His Boldness, 156. *See also* Lake, John G.
Johnson, Milbank, 132
Juice fasting, 28. *See also* Detoxification; Fasting

K

Karnstedt, James, 46
Kaznachayev, V.F., 134
Kendall, Arthur I, 133
King David, 126
King James, 1, 21, 53, 85, 97, 105, 139, 183
King James Bible, 1, 21, 53, 85, 105, 139, 183
King Solomon, 152, 164
Kingdom of Heaven, 2-20, 139, 142, 146, 157-169,174-177, 181, 197. *See also* Heavenly Kingdom
Knights Templar, 97
Koch, William Frederick, 101
Koch Treatment, 101
Krebs (tricarboxylic acid) cycle, 108

L

Lactic acid, 50; build up, 45
Lactobacillus acidophilus, 25
Lake, John G., 163. *See also* the book *John G. Lake: His Life, His Sermons, His Boldness*
Language, words and Spirit, 130. *See also* God's words
Laser light, 136
Law of contact, 160
Law of Divine judgement, 175. *See also* God
Laxatives, 44
Levi priests, 121, 124. *See also* L'vi'im
Lifestyle risks, 47
Light refraction, 131
Lipoic acid, 73
Lips, 140; lying abomination, 159; powerful creative force for health, 140. *See also* Words
Lissajous, Jules-Antoine, 115
Litton Bionetics, 191

Negative air ions, 104
Negative Population Growth, Inc. of New Jersey, 92. *See also* Rockefeller family; population control
Nettle leaf, 34
New covenant, 99. *See also* Covenant
New York City Blood Council, 92, 95. *See also* Rockefeller family; population control
Nutritional Supplements for Immunity, Energy, Acuity, Rest and Recovery, 53, 59. *See also* Immune system

O

Oat bran, 28
Oates, David John , 125
Optimal health, 38
Organ transplants, 55
Organic produce, 57
Organochlorines, 46
Overeating, 20
Oxidizing pathogenic microbes, 88. *See also* Oxygenation
Oxygenation(therapies), 5, 20, 21, 32, 34, 41, 85, 87-95, 100-106

P

Panax Ginseng, 34
Pau d'arco, 29, 37
Paul, the Apostle, 4; Divine counsel, 129
Peace, 3, 20, 20, 89, 93, 109, 128, 140, 163, 166-168, 176
pH, 37-47, 50, 88. *See also* Body chemistry
Pharmaceutical industry, 2; propaganda, 2
Photon energy, 135
Photon-phonon emissions, 109; transduction, 111
Physics of sound, 163. *See also* sound.
Phytonutrients, 57
Piezoelectric interactions, 111
Poiesz, Bernard J. , 90
Polished rice, 53
Pooling human blood, 187
Population control, 55, 94, 190. *See also* Rockefeller family; Merck Fund
Positive feedback, 20. *See also* Cybernetics
Potassium chloride, 43
Potassium iodide, 71
Power of language, 120. *See also* Sound; Word; Reverse speech
Prana, 98

Prayer and healing, 163. *See also* Miracles; Words; Electromagnetics of sound
Predestination, 20
Preparing Your Temple of God: The End Times Sermon, 53
Preservatives, 22
Pressman, A.S., 113
Price, Weston, 49
Project EISCAT, 136
Project HAARP, 136
Propolis extract, 71
Prostate glands, 51
Provisions, 170. *See also* tithing
Psyllium husks, 22, 25. *See also* Flora Fit™
Pythagorean mathematics, 56; skein, 119, 121, 122

Q

Quantum physics, 56
Quartz, 134; crystal, 134. *See also* Electromagnetics; Electromedicine; Clustered water

R

Racial Hygiene Society, 188. *See also* IG Farben; Rockefeller family
Radio frequencies, 132. *See also* Sound; Electromagnetics
Raise the dead, 140. *See also* Miracles
Rape oil, 77. *See also* Canola oil
Ray, William, 47
Red blood cells, 98
Refined carbohydrates, 53
Relationships, 146; based on trust, 146. *See also* Trust
Report From Iron Mountain, 137
Respiratory distress, 76. *See also* Flu-like illness
Respiratory system, 33, 34
Retinyl-palmitate, 62
Reverse osmosis, 46
Reverse speech, 125. *See also* Oates, David John
Rheumatoid arthritis, 60
Rife, Royal Raymond, 105, 131-133
Righteousness, 2, 20, 20, 146, 163, 164, 175
Rockefeller famly, 93, 192; directed blood banking industry, 91; Foundation, 94, 192; monopolized American medicine, 91
Rockefeller, Laurance, 95. *See also* Rockefeller family
Rosa canina, 33

Vibrational medicine, 133; see also *Electromedicine*.
Vibratory essence of Spirit, 130. *See also* Electromagnetics
Victory over afflictions, 151. *See also* Miracles
Viola odorata, 33
Violet leaves, 33
Viral infections, 38, 136. see also *Viruses*.
Viruses, 4, 22, 25, 38, 50, 55, 58, 60, 64, 70, 76, 77, 82, 87, 89, 91, 94, 95, 98, 105, 131, 132, 136, 182, 186-188, 192
Vitamin A, 61, 62, 65, 67
Vitamin C, 33, 34, 69, 70, 73, .88
Vitamin E, 73, 74

W

Wainwright, Basil, 86
Warburg, Otto, 89
Water 44, 109, 165; clusters, 165; for hydration, 44; molecules, 109; molecular structure of, 108. *See also* Clustered water
Watermelon fasts, 28. *See also* Detoxification; Fasting
Western diet, 39
White blood cells, 69, 98, 186
White flour, 53
Wholistic approach, 21
Wisdom of Solomon, 1, 2. *See also* Solomon, King
Winter, Dan, 116
Word of Adonai, 154. *See also* God; Bible.
Words from the Lips, 163. *See also* Lips; Sound; Spoken word
World Health Organization, 107

X

X-ray radiation, 67

Y

Yeast, 25, 135, 186
Yeshua, 3, 5, 20, 20, 20, 96, 99, 107, 109, 124, 126, 130, 139, 142, 146, 157-169, 175-181, 197; His blood, 96. *See also* Jesus

Z

Zinc chelate, 35

About the Author

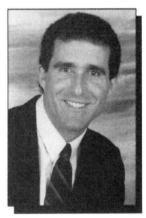 Leonard G. Horowitz, D.M.D., M.A., M.P.H., is a Harvard graduate, an internationally known authority in public health and AIDS education, and one of healthcare's most captivating motivational speakers. He earned his doctorate in medical dentistry from Tufts University, a master of arts degree in health education from Beacon College, and a master of public health degree in behavioral science from Harvard University.

Dr. Horowitz has served on the faculties of Tufts University, Harvard University, and Leslie College's Institute for the Arts and Human Development. He has also served as a consultant to several leading healthcare corporations, national associations, and academic institutions.

Dr. Horowitz has authored over one hundred articles, and more than two dozen books, videotapes and audiocassette health programs including the critically acclaimed best-seller, *Emerging Viruses: AIDS & Ebola—Nature, Accident or Intentional?*, and *Healing Codes for the Biological Apocalypse*. This latter work won him "Author of the Year Award" by the World Natural Health Organization in 1999. In addition, his work in vaccine risk awareness, particularly with the publication of the bestselling audiotape *Horowitz "On Vaccines,"* and the videotape *Emerging Viruses and Vaccinations*, has gained him international recognition and praise by leaders of several Third World nations.

Dr. Horowitz is a Christian (Messianic) Jew who consistently expresses a heightened sense of spirituality in his personal and professional life. A loving husband and father of three children, he spends his free time hiking, skiing, sailing, swimming, snorkeling, and singing.

Diary/Notes

Notes

Notes

Notes

Tetrahedron

Health science communications

for people around the world

Publishing Group

Catalog of Books, Tapes and Health Products
Call 1-888-508-4787 9am - 5pm PST

NEW!!!

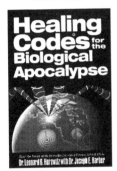

"A pleasure to read and study. . . . A phenomenal work by two truly remarkable humanitarieans. Five stars ☆ ☆ ☆ ☆ ☆" — *WNHO Endorsement Magazine*

One half of the world's current population should soon be dead according to authorita tive projections. Will you, your family and friends be among the survivors or the deceased?

Dr. Len Horowitz and Dr. Joseph Barber investigate 2000 years of religious and political persecution and the latest technologies being used to enslave, coerce and even kill billions of unsuspecting people.

This work returns the most precious spiritual knowledge, power and "healing codes" to humanity. It offers new hope for the loving masses to survive the worldwide plagues, famine and weather changes that are now at hand. In perfect time for these cataclysmic events, *Healing Codes* presents an urgent, monumental, and inspired work that will be hailed for generations to come.

517 Page HardcoverBook $26.95

Bestselling Book!

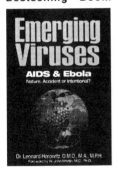

"Shocking. The boldest of new books of alternative medicine."
— *Alternative Medicine Digest*

This is the first in-depth exploration into the origins of the AIDS and Ebola viruses. Claims that these "emerging viruses" naturally evolved and then jumped species from monkey to man are grossly unfounded in light of the compelling evidence assembled in this extraordinary text. Alternatively, the possibility that these bizarre germs were laboratory creations, accidentally or intentionally transmitted via tainted vaccines in the U.S. and Africa, is documented here.

The accidental and genocidal theories of AIDS are meticuously explored within the social and political context of this stormy period of American military science. The text hauntingly dissects the potential motives and administrative mechanisms underlying the prevalent belief that HIV and Ebola were deliberately deployed.

592 Page Hardcover Book $29.95
3 Hour Audio $19.95
2 1/2 Hour Video $29.95

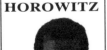
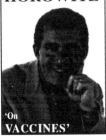

Horowitz 'On Vaccines'—Bestselling Audio

If you have questions about the safety and efficacy of vaccines then this tape is for you. How effective are vaccines? What risks do they pose? Why have so many vaccines suddenly become required? Are they truly "mandated by law," and if not, how can you and your children exempt from vaccine programs if so desired? This tape explains how vaccines are delivering AIDS, chronic fatigue, many types of cancer, Gulf War Syndrome and a host of autoimmune diseases including fibromyalgia, MS, lupus, Guillain Barre, asthma, allergies, autism and even hyperactivity and attention deficit disorders.

90 Minute Audio $14.95

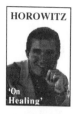

Horowitz on Healing - NEW!!!

Reviews the critical five steps required to defend against the current and coming plagues. These includ 1) detoxification, 2) deacidification, 3) boosting immunity, 4) oxygenation therapies, and 5) bioelectr therapies. These recommendations are especially beneficial for people who are ailing with auto-immur disorders and cancer.

90 Minute Audio $14.9

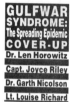

GulfWar Syndrome: The Spreading Epidemic Cover-up

Gulf War Syndrome, an infectious disease related to biological warfare, contaminate vaccines and chronic fatigue, affects more than 200,000 veterans and is spreading rapidl to civilian populations. As the CIA and Pentagon spreads disinformation and doubt, children, health profes sionals and even pets are becoming infected, ill and are dying. This video presents th unnerving truth, documented facts, and urgently needed help for millions of people worldwide who ar rightfully concerned about this spreading plague.

3 1/2 Hour Video $24.9

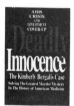

Deadly Innocence—The Kimberly Bergalis Case

Dr. Horowitz reads his critically acclaimed book that exposes the Centers for Disease Control and Preventio (CDC) for covering up virtually all of the incriminating evidence against the Florida dentist responsible fo infecting Kimberly Bergalis and at least five other patients with the AIDS virus. Learn what Dr. Acer wa really like, how his personality profile matched those of thirty-six serial killers studied by the FBI, why h committed serial homicide, and why the government investigators covered up the evidence to leave the case a "unsolvable mystery."

3 Hour Audio $19.9
2 Hour Video $24.9

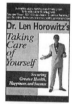

Taking Care of Yourself—Boosting Immunity

Optimal health, happiness and success are yours to enjoy by following the breakthrough step detailed here by public health education authority, Dr. Len Horowitz. This interactiv audio and guidebook package provides easy to follow instructions to succeed in your quest for powerfu immunity against common illnesses and the coming plagues. By making Dr. Horowitz's common sens recommendations part of your daily routine, you might even save your life and others will love and appre ciate you more! Includes the Nutritional Supplements, Horowitz on Healing and Survival Water, pH anc Oxygen tape sets listed below.

9 Hour Audio Program with Workbook $69.95

The Nazi–American Biomedical/Biowarfare Connection

If you think the Nazi agenda for world control, disposing of undesirable populations, and experiments to genetically develop a master race ended with World War II, you are in for a shocker! Learn how Hitler's top medical and biowarfare researchers served U.S. and British intelligence, allied pharmaceutical and population control interests, along with the Rockefellers, the Bushes and the British Royal Family!

3 Hour Audio $19.95

Virus Makers of the CIA

Join Dr. Horowitz and three other experts in biowarfare research, vaccine contamination and U. S. Government cover-ups, as they are interviewed by nationally syndicated radio talk show host Dave Emory. These heroic authors discuss the most controversial and horrifying facts about the current and coming plagues including why we now have epidemics of cancer, AIDS, Ebola, chronic fatigue, Gulf War Syndrome and more. This tape is absolutely rivoting!

3 Hour Audio $19.95

Call 1-888-508-4787 9am - 5pm PST

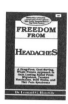

Freedom From Headaches

This package provides a complete selfcare program to help diagnose, treat, and prevent headaches.

90 Min. Audio & 72 Pg. Book
$14.95

Freedom From Teeth Clenching

This program will put you to sleep fast and will help you to stop the unhealthy habit of night grinding.

60 Min. Audio & 32 Pg. Book
$14.95

Freedom From Dental Anxiety

This package contains all that you need to conquer debilitating dental fears at an extremely affordable price.

90 Min. Audio & 20 Pg. Book
$19.95

Freedom From Job Stress

This complete guide will help you improve your workstation, office environment and personal habits to keep you healthy, happy and more productive.

60 Min. Audio & 70 Pg. Book
$14.95

- INTERVIEWS BY DR. HOROWITZ -

Survival Water: pH and Oxygen - NEW!!!

Your body is more than eighty percent water and if you're not drinking the right kind of water you may be in trouble. Not only is water contamination a potential problem, but the pH and oxygenation levels of the water largely determine your health or disease status. Eliminate the guesswork and learn from Jim Karnstedt, a leading authority on water, pH and oxygenation therapies, as he is interviewed by Dr. Len Horowitz.

90 Minute Audio   **$14.95**

Nutritional Supplements for Immunity, Energy, Acuity and more

Dr. Horowitz interviews nutritional supplement expert James South about boosting immunity and energy and recovering from cancer, chronic fatigue and more. Learn how nutritional supplements are combined to act synergistically with your immune system and how vitamins, minerals, herbs and hormones can work to improve your health. The latest advances in nutritional science can be practically applied by you in your selection and use of supplements to improve mental acuity, boost energy, and induce restful and healing sleep.

3 Hour Audio   **$19.95**

Why It's Time Jews and Christians Unite

Was the bible revised to create the rift between Christians and Jews? Dr. Weinstein, interviewed by Dr. Horowitz, has convincing arguments to show: the vast majority of Jews, at the time of Christ, believed Jesus was their Messiah; Jesus's message was distorted to foment unrest and separation between Christians and Jews; and Jews were falsely accused of causing the death of Jesus.

3 Hour Audio   **$19.95**

End Times: Preparedness, Prophecy & Propaganda — NEW!

Dr. Len Horowitz proudly presents an interview with Pastor Norm Franz—one of the nation's leading experts on bible prophecy. On this new audiotape, the two educators discuss the most important issues of our time including how to: prepare for the great shaking or tribulation and the messianic age; understand "alien" phenomena; and see through the "New World Order" and its spiritual implications.

90 Minute Audio   **$14.95**

Call 1-888-508-4787   9am - 5pm PST

Order Form   Call 1-888-508-4787   (7:30am - 4:30pm PST)
[order 24 hours daily on our secure website and save 10%: www.tetrahedron.org]

Name _____   Order Date _____

Phone # _____   Where did you hear about us? _____

Address: _____   Billing Information: ☐ Visa ☐ MasterCard ☐ Check

_____   Account # _____

_____   Expiration Date _____

ORDER QUANTITIES OF BOOKS AND TAPES AND SAVE!!!	5 OR MORE OF ONE TITLE . . . . 20% DISCOUNT 10 OR MORE OF ONE TITLE . . . . . . 40% DISCOUNT 16 OR MORE OF ONE TITLE . . . . . . 50% DISCOUNT

TITLE	QTY.	COST	TOTAL
Christianity Unmasqued		$21.95	
Deadly Innocence: The Bergalis Case - Audio		$19.25*	
Death In The Air - Book		$29.15*	
" "Live" Video Presentation		$39.50*	
" "Live" Audio Presentation		$19.25*	
Divine Harmony Music - CD		$19.25	
Emerging Viruses: AIDS and Ebola - Book		$29.15*	
" "Live" Video Presentation		$29.15*	
" "Live" Audio Presentation		$19.25*	
End Times Prophecy Audio		$14.75	
Freedom From Desk Job Stress . . . Audio		$14.75	
Freedom From Dental Anxiety Audio		$19.25	
Freedom From Headaches Audio		$14.75	
Freedom From Teeth Clenching . . . Audio		$14.75	
Gulf War Syndrome: The Spreading Epidemic Coverup Video		$24.65*	
Healing Celebrations - Book		$22.85*	
" "Live" Audio Presentation		$39.50*	
" "Live" Video Presentation		$39.50*	
Healing Codes for the Biological Apocalypse-Book		$26.45*	
" "Live" Video Presentation		$39.50*	
" "Live" Audio Presentation		$24.65	
Healing Tones - CD		$15.65	
Healing Tones - Audio		$12.50	
Holy Harmony CD		$16.55	
Horowitz 'on Healing' Audio		$14.75	
Horowitz 'on Vaccines' Audio		$14.75*	
Jewish Bible - Hard Cover		$39.50	
Jewish Bible - Soft Cover		$32.75	
Lost Chord CD		$16.55	
Nazi-American Bio medical warfare Connection Audio		$19.25*	
Preparing the Temple of God		$14.75	
Survival Water: pH and Oxygen Audio		$14.75	
Taking Care of Yourself Package		$48.50*	
Virus Makers of the CIA: Biowar Forum Audio		$19.25*	
Why It's Time Jews & Christians Unite Audio		$24.65	

Books & Tapes Shipping and Handling:			
First Item	$5.30	Subtotal	
Each Additional Item	$1.70	Shipping & Handling	
International Orders Add	$5.00 extra		
Each Additional International Item Add	$2.00 extra		
Priority Mail Add	$2.00	TOTAL	

PACKAGE SPECIALS	QTY	COST	TOTAL
One of Everything with * - (Save $51.80)		$350.00 S&H $29.10	
4 Book Special - (Save $18.60) Emerging Viruses: AIDS & Ebola Healing Codes for the Biological Apocalypse Healing Celebrations Death in the Air		$89.00 S&H $10.40	
5 Audiocassette Special - (Save $23.90) Emerging Viruses and Vaccinations Healing Codes for the Biological Apocalypse Healing Celebrations Horowitz on Vaccines Horowitz on Healing		$89.00 S&H $9.00	
Emerging Viruses Special - (Save $13.15) Emerging Viruses: AIDS & Ebola-book Emerging Viruses and Vaccinations-video Horowitz on Vaccines-audiotape		$60.00 S&H $8.70	
Healing Codes Special - (Save $20.70) Healing Codes for the Biological Apocalypse-book Healing Codes for the Biological Apocalypse-video Horowitz on Healing-audiotape		$60.00 S&H $8.70	
Death in the Air Special - (Save $13.15) Death in the Air-book Emerging Viruses and Vaccinations-video Horowitz on Healing-audiotape		$60.00 S&H $8.70	
Taking Care of Yourself Special - (Save $22.50) Healing Celebrations-book Taking Care of Yourself package		$70.00 S&H $8.70	
Celebrations Educational Package- (Save $109.55) Healing Celebrations-book Healing Celebrations-video Healing Celebrations-audio Taking Care of Yourself package Divine Harmony-CD The Lost Chord-CD Death in the Air-book Horowitz on Vaccines-audiotape		$152.00 S&H $8.70	

**Contact us with any change of address,
to update our mailing list and receive our newsletters.
Please allow 7-21 business days for delivery**

HEALTHY WORLD DISTRIBUTING
206 North 4th Avenue, Suite 147 · Sandpoint, ID 83864 · 208-265-2575 · Fax: 208-265-2775 · www.tetrahedron.org